HOMEOPATHY,
s w e e t
HOMEOPATHY

coming home to perfect health

Pierre Fontaine RSHom CCH

ISBN: 1-4392-1964-8
ISBN-13: 9781439219645

Visit www.booksurge.com to order additional copies.

Dedication.

To *mon Papa* who suffered from illnesses most of his life and to my sister Francoise who didn't live long enough.

Giving Thanks

The one person I can thank the most for this book is Craig, a beautiful soul. Craig put a lot of time and effort in this project and had the sensitivity to surprise me with compliments right after reading my first draft. I cannot thank him enough.

More particularly, I thank all the people who put their trust in homeopaths all around the world and help us fine tune this brilliantly effective healing art. I bow before those who taught me and extend my admiration to those who make the system of homeopathy ever more effective, they are my heroes.

Thank you to my mother, who provided me with great freedom and unlimited trust. She taught me to speak my mind because she doesn't know any other way! I also thank my whole wonderful family in France who always provided me with the warmest welcome; I am grateful to them for their generosity.

Thanks to my wife Carolina who stuck by me, and without whom I could not have been as clear as I am in this book. Every sentence has a little bit of her. Gloriana and Florencia, my two daughters who give me a sense that I may be a good dad, I don't know.

And finally to Providence and the Earth for I have no idea why I was born where I was born but I sure like it.

Thank you all so much.

Pierre Fontaine RSHom CCH
New York, NY
October 2008

TABLE OF CONTENTS

PART II

38 CASES FROM MY PRACTICE

A NOTE

I have a special place in my heart for Autism Spectrum Disorder (ASD) kids, a disorder I am proud to have taken a very special interest in for many years. I poured myself into these kids. At times, I thought I was holding a good key to improve their condition but in the long run the results spoke for themselves and they were not up to what I expected from homeopathy. It seemed like a tortuous journey, I never despaired and then I began to write this book. While going back through my cases, I noticed that the children who were doing exceptionally well had one thing in common. It was a Eureka! moment. The apple had fallen and all I needed to do was unravel what had fallen in my lap. At this point, I have just about unraveled the whole thing and most of the children improve enormously. It will be the main subject of my second book, "Homeopathy Sweet Homeopathy. Autism, PDD-NOS, Asperger's, Dyspraxia, Apaxia: The Journey Back Home Unraveled."

For this book, I wanted to give these children a front row seat. I asked two mothers, Mary Hernandez and Fatos Yuruk to write about their experiences with their children and homeopathy. I asked them to write whatever is on their mind and in their hearts, confident that their words would be better than anything I can say.

As it turns out, each wrote in a very different style mimicking the duality of part two of this book. Mary's foreword relates to the way I consult for children now. The results tend to be crisp and sharp. On the other hand, Fatos writes about her experience with homeopathy before I made a series of breakthroughs that help solve the problem altogether.

Enjoy.

Foreword 1

by Maria Hernandez, son diagnosed with autism:

I just want to say that Pierre has made an amazing difference with my son in removing his autism diagnosis. With DAN! (Defeat Autism Now!) doctors and other therapies (believe me, we have been through *so* many) my son was a good responder, but he was still autistic and we suffered a number of severe regressions that sent him back into severe autism. I knew even though he went from very severe at age 4 to relatively high functioning, that the situation was very tenuous and fragile. I visited Pierre Fontaine and he recommended a remedy for my son. He has so rapidly lost his remaining autistic characteristics that I am in a state of shock every day. Rather than therapies and managing autism, I now find myself rushing to keep up with education to fill in the gaps. He is a child who at 9 is suddenly motivated to socialize and make friends, though he has a lot of learning to do to catch up, he is doing it so fast! He has such an amazing new awareness of the difference between himself and other kids with autism. I heard him explain to a neighbor child the other day when a friend's child was over (who is very similar to how Luis used to be), "I can't come over to play today because there is a boy who has autism at my house and I need to help my mom take care of him. He doesn't understand a lot of things. I have autism too, but I understand a lot of things now." It was the first time this boy stayed at our house that I was able to do other things besides monitor him as my son told me, "Don't worry, Mom. You can do your work. I'll take care of Justin. I understand him. He's like I used to be." Of course, I had to leave the room because I was crying tears of joy. And he did a great job playing with Justin and keeping him in line. (Justin has a lot of negative behaviors...) My son said to me the other night, "Maybe soon I won't have any more autism."

I have to admit I saw nothing with the first dose of the remedy and was thinking that maybe this Pierre was a fraud or just not knowledgeable. (We had been to a classical homeopath before who charged us a fortune and did nothing.) But with the second water dose of the remedy Pierre recommended last January we went from severe aggression and tantrums that required restraining my son for a minimum of 1-2 hours a day to NO tantrums or aggression whatsoever. Since then it has just been getting better every day from there. He doesn't have any issues with mainstreaming now and is in the moment and attentive pretty much all the time. And if he starts to daydream he catches himself. "Hey Mom, I spaced out there for a minute...." I cannot tell you how this has so dramatically changed our life as a family.

Thank you to Pierre!!!!

Mary

Foreword 2

by Mrs Fatos Yuruk, son diagnosed with PDD-NOS:

Our son was diagnosed with PDD-NOS at the age of two years and two months. We immediately researched it on the Internet and started him on GF/CF diet and started seeing some changes in only a few days. We increased speech therapy sessions, started him on ABA therapy, OT, PT, Speech Prompt therapy. Our DAN! doctor tried to impose a diabetes drug he had been testing on autistic kids and his pediatrician only prescribed a multi-vitamin with added fluoride. These "treatments" did not satisfy us.

Our son was a happy, social and vocal infant though he always had a cough and a runny nose while teething. He met all his milestones until he was 18 months when we noticed some speech delay. He was 22 months when he lost his vocabulary and eye contact.

We decided to give homeopathy a six-month trial after reading Amy Lansky's book on homeopathy and her son's recovery of autism. Amy forwarded me a few homeopath referrals in the NYC area. Pierre Fontaine was the first to pick up the phone so our journey began. Before seeing him we traded e-mails, he wanted us to write about our son; his likes, dislikes anything about him other than autistic traits. When we met, Deniz had already made great progress cognitively with different therapies but he was still a non-verbal, under-reactive boy with a great attention span to put together 48 piece interlocking puzzles, typing and knowing letters, shapes, the alphabet and reading. He was also sick very often.

Thuja was the first remedy we tried. May 8th was the first dose, we waited 2-3 days and on May 11th we gave a second dose. He coughed at 3 am with a dry cough at night, wet cough during the day and lots of nasal discharge. In a few days he started visual stimming [stimulating]. On May 26th we repeated a dose, he woke up sticking his tongue out and moved it much more easily, his speech therapist had been working on this for months with no luck. He became much more aware of his surroundings. We were witnessing good results and we thought something was working. However as he became more aware, stimming increased. It was extremely nerve-racking for us. He had some gains but he looked much more autistic. Mr. Fontaine said it was a way for kids to overcome the anxiety that may be caused by increased awareness. Stimming decreased and disappeared in 2 months.

In July, Mr. Fontaine suggested we give him red clay bath. After the second bath he had bad rash on his face, which cleared up in 2 days. We observed an increase in his connection with us. He was slowly improving but every 2-3 weeks, he would get a dry cough. Mr. Fontaine gave him the homeopathic remedy *Mercurius solubilis*. He took a long nap after taking it and stopped coughing. His speech kept improving. He started talking.

On November 25, 2007, he had bronchitis and an ear infection. It started with a cough and a gag upon hearing about food. For a few days he didn't eat except for rice milk and gluten-free cookies. On the 26th and 28th he had low-grade fever at night and vomited a few times during the day. On Nov. 29th the doctor diagnosed him with an ear infection in his left ear and bronchitis and was prescribed Albuterol and Augmentin. She mentioned the side effect of Albuterol: hyperactivity. We were torn between giving a homeopathy a shot and waiting a day to get the remedy or go to the pharmacy and get what the doctor prescribed. We waited for an uncommon remedy... We gave *Mercurius cyanatus* 30C on Nov. 30 and Dec. 1st. Gagging upon hearing of food was a clear and distinguishing symptom according to Pierre. It stopped after the first dose, his appetite increased and the coughing stopped. In only two days he got better. That week we noticed a jump in his cognitive and communication skills. Our follow-up visit with the pediatrician was on Monday, Dec. 10 and she said to discontinue the antibiotics - we didn't tell her about homeopathy. He did not have an infection anymore. She also said he had recovered from bronchitis. We used this remedy whenever he gagged on food.

On February 29th flu-like symptoms started in the evening. After dinner he developed a low-grade fever with watery and itchy eyes. We gave "FluCare for Kidz." He was active and playful, by 7PM he fell asleep waking up every few hours coughing. We tried to control the symptoms by using other remedy cocktails for a few days but he didn't get better. We called Pierre Fontaine who recommended *Euphrasia* during our phone consultation. It worked like a miracle, after one dose on March 6th he slept for 17 hours. He woke up to drink some water and rice milk and went back to sleep. Then he woke up feeling better on Sunday morning.

This showed us how a single remedy can work quickly when precisely given. Only one dose of *Euphrasia* did the trick for him to get better.

In April Mr. Fontaine explained he had come to some breakthroughs regarding the treatment of children. After my appointment with Mr. Fontaine another remedy picture emerged: *Rubidium Carbonicum*. Deniz has been on this remedy for the last 6 months on an "as needed" basis.

Deniz is now 4 years old with a wide range of vocabulary with interest in math, music, books, and soccer. He expresses his needs clearly, has great connection with us, and his eye contact is steadily improving. His interaction with other kids is emerging. His appetite is still not great - he eats variety of veggies, meat and rice but is very picky when it comes to fruits. He still gets sick and as winter approaches we're keeping an eye on any new patterns that may indicate a new remedy picture.

Above are our success stories since we started using homeopathy in the last 18 months. It's very challenging to find the perfect match to your symptoms but when found it's effective yet gentle. It's all about observing the symptoms, taking notes and figuring out the pattern.

Medications are not safe for our kids. It's wonderful to have homeopathy with no side effects and such healing power.

Mrs. Fatos Yuruk

Foreword

This book is a new concept in homeopathic books inasmuch as it presents a wide array of actual cases to the general public. Ever since Doctor Samuel Hahnemann began to formulate the system of homeopathy 200 years ago, but first spoken of by Hippocrates, it has always let its cases speak for themselves. The innumerable professional books are replete with cases of all kinds but they are indented for the professional homeopath who understands the finer intricacies of this remedial science.

People seek a professional homeopath mainly because friends, partners or acquaintances have described how much better they feel. That's great, but what I often hear is this: "I tell everybody about homeopathy but they don't understand what it is that you do. It seems too strange and it is so difficult to explain."

So here it is. *Homeopathy, Sweet Homeopathy* is meant to answer these questions and give the people a sense of what it is, what it can do, how it works and how it should be practiced.

You will find 33 different conditions out of 38 different cases from acne to Lupus and Crohn's disease to Post Traumatic Stress Disorder. Each case and its discussion can be read independently of the other cases. Each case speaks about the disorder as a totality of physical and emotional symptoms as well as to the experience associated to one's illness. The discussion speaks to the rationale or logic of homeopathy. The reader will understand enough of the homeopathic approach to get a deep sense of what is for most people an enigmatic health profession.

Homeopathy, Sweet Homeopathy presents the human life experience of being sick and the return at its high of being healthy. I sincerely hope you can find comfort in the fact there are options and that homeopathy can effectively and safely help you and your loved one overcome health concerns whether these have been long- or short-term.

Enjoy.

Pierre Fontaine RSHom CCH
Classical Homeopath
315 W 57th St., Suite 308
New York, NY 10019
(212) 334-7360
www.homeopathicservices.com

The highest ideal of cure is the rapid, gentle and permanent restoration of health in the least disadvantageous way.

Samuel Hahneman

INTRODUCTION

With this book you find yourself in my consultation room; you are peeking in, hearing* and watching what is going on. It is like being invited backstage; you become a witness to the process of restoring health in a wholesome, most effective and natural manner.

This book is about human stories, people's illnesses with which some of you will surely identify. You will find yourself saying "Oh, that sounds like me!" or "I think so and so has this," or even, "Oh, that's crazy!" This is good because the point here is that all these cases are about life, how it is affected by illness and how illness can be reversed with homeopathy. In contrast, I have never heard anyone say, "Oh, I have the same blood test as yours!" and get excited about it; that is because there is no life there, just some numbers and a foreign word as a conclusion.

I think when people visit a homeopath they want someone who has the knowledge to understand the web of symptoms, disorders and more importantly can make sense of the inter-relatedness from which they suffer as a whole. Most people think one problem they are suffering from in their body is somehow related to another - it is instinctual - but the medical system does not affirm that. The intuition of the interconnectivity of ailments and symptoms is already, from the point of the homeopath, a much deeper understanding of one's condition than the doctor will ever know. Indeed, the sense of relatedness is right. You will see the proof of alleviating suffering in totality over and over again in these cases.

Each case begins with a list of complaints. First, a main complaint (MC); underneath MC is a list of other complaints because there is rarely just one pain or one issue bothering people. Once people see the process of the homeopathic consultation, they realize they might as well tell me about the rest of their complaints.

The relationships between the different conditions and disorders are what I call the "golden thread." The golden thread weaves the disorders together within the person. It is also what leads to the best remedy in a logical manner, thereby resolving all the ailments at once. This is the exceptional beauty of homeopathy. Instead of treating the different parts it gives us the tools to lift all at once. Think about it! How could the parts of you be treated without the whole of you? Arthritis, Lupus, Irritable Bowel Syndrome (IBS), don't walk in the office. You, with your health problems, walk into the office. When you treat the parts, or the different diagnoses separately which is what happens when you take different medications, you end up with something that is not quite health. By interfering or antagonizing the natural process with suppressive agents you end up with different biological processes that are actually not quite you.

Talking about illness and its effects in the body and on life is fascinating but talking about healing is far more exciting. To hear people say they feel better than ever before as a whole is not only rewarding to me but it is also fantastic for my clients. "I didn't know I could feel so good." That's beautiful to hear. When people say they "feel better" it is not only because they no longer have the physical symptoms they were suffering from before but also because of freedom gained on emotional and mental level. This translates to the marriage being saved because the person is no longer affected by a disorder clouding the mind and now does not see the problems that existed the same way anymore. There is a larger reality. It is not only the migraine that is gone as in Tom's case, it is also the obsession about neatly setting up the ingredients in ramekins prior to cooking as if it were a cooking show that is gone.

This is the real human story, the duality of disease and its effects on people. The beauty of homeopathy is its ability to understand illness within the context of the individual story in a way that makes total sense. From that "total sense" - what homeopaths call the *totality* - a remedy is recommended that will lead to a complete alleviation of suffering. We are a long way from Petri dishes, blood tests and machines that shoot rays, pulsate or radiate to alter the course of diseases. We are in the heart of human disorder rather than merely in the midst of technology.

This case-illustrated book is guaranteed to fascinate even the most skeptical of skeptics. These cases speak to the value of homeopathy rather than making an argument for or against it. You can make up your mind with real life concrete examples. It is not my goal to argue whether homeopathy works or not. It works and you see it. If anyone wants to argue against homeopathy, I say, "Don't argue with me, argue with the people who feel better and convince them that they actually are not!"

The orthodox establishment tells us, "Prove to me that it works." My answer to that is very simple. "No, I don't have to prove anything." We all know that no matter what or how many times we prove homeopathy works through well-designed studies and cases, some will never believe it. This is the way the world works and it is just fine by me since I am not here to persuade anyone. Those who come to homeopathy come for different reasons:

1. It makes sense to them
2. It is effective

3. They are tired of taking different medications they feel do not get rid of the problems, but rather mask them

4. It is as harmless as it can be

I am often told, "You don't believe in medicine." I also hear the following statement, "I don't believe in homeopathy." When people say this to me I say tongue-in-cheek, "I don't believe in homeopathy either." That generally takes my interlocutor by surprise but the fact is I don't believe in homeopathy at all nor do I want to believe in it. If I did, it would not reflect on me well. To me, it simply works. It is not a belief, it is a fact. This is a certainty and because of that I practice it. That is all that matters to me. The rest is baggage I do not need to carry. It goes back to the argument of proving it. I don't need to please everyone (which is not possible anyway). I do want to please those who are interested. Homeopathy and medicine, for that matter, are not religions. You don't need to believe in either one. It baffles me to hear that. I don't think anyone should make a decision about health and disease on whether one believes in anything.

I am not against conventional medicine; some of my best friends are doctors! There is a difference between the two systems and each thinks that his way is better according to the information each one has at his disposal. That said, what I consistently find is that the information the "non-believers" have is at best very limited. When a doctor tells me, "I don't believe in homeopathy," I usually ask whether he has ever been to a homeopathic conference. The answer is always "No!" There are mountains of studies that prove homeopathy to be effective. I am just not interested in debating them. Statistics bore me and I imagine bore you, too; I am much more interested in life. Besides, anyone can make anything out statistics. So this book is meant to inform you based on the process of what we do in the consultation room. It offers an optimistic solution for your health and I hope you enjoy it.

* There is a small caveat to this. Some of the questions I ask during consultation are transcribed here but the repetition of them is not nearly the same as it is written. At times I ask the same question over and over and over again in order to come through different levels to reach a deeper understanding. To make reading more pleasant I had to limit and edit some of the consultations to a minimum.

In the healthy human state, the life force that enlivens the body keeps all parts of the organism in a harmonious state of operation, as regards both feelings and functions, so that our indwelling, rational spirit can freely avail itself of this living, healthy instrument for the higher purposes of our existence.

Samuel Hahnemann

CHAPTER 1

HOMEOPATHY EXPLAINED

Homeopathy is a biodynamic alternative to the biochemical medicine model we know.

Biodynamic simply means we recognize that something animates and keeps us alive. If a Being is not alive it is dead! There is no in between here. The question then is: What keeps us alive? A lot of people say the soul. To me, the soul is a spiritual entity attached or connected to God in the same sense that a grain of sand is connected to the earth. The soul is potentially pure Godly energy and therefore is not directly related to homeopathy. Medicine, alternative medicine, acupuncture or homeopathy do not have anything to do with that directly. There is so much talk about the spiritual in the alternative field in my opinion that the word has become skewed in meaning. There is nothing spiritual about a massage, for example. It feels good and it may be relaxing. But spiritual? I don't think so. So let's not get confused, restoring health on the physical, emotional and mental level is a tall enough order without getting into the dicey, dogmatic and personal spirituality that is between you, your conscience and whatever you believe.

Most homeopaths call what keeps us alive "the Vital Force" (VF) or "the *dynamis*." The Vital Force has a different purpose than the soul. The Vital Force is the bridge between the spiritual i.e. the soul, and the realization or phenomenon of life into the material body. It is like an umbilical cord between the soul and the physical body. There is no abrupt break between any of them. One could say the soul does not need a Vital Force unless it wants to manifest in the physical world. On the other hand, the Vital Force doesn't exist without a soul. The Vital Force is subservient to the soul, yet the soul does not dictate to the Vital Force; it is far too wise to do so. To put it in a simple way, the soul is like a car and the Vital Force is like the driver. The car does not need a driver to be a car but in order to go somewhere it needs a driver. The driver is the one who acts either as a great driver or a reckless one. They do form an indispensable unit to each other to fulfill the purpose of a car. This elementary analogy holds true in many different ways in the body, at the cellular level in the transcription of DNA in the cellular nucleus to RNA, which then travels outside the nucleus into the cytoplasm. In short, since something keeps us alive it stands to reason that it must be essential in the process of health.

The concept of vitality is really a very familiar one, albeit a forgotten one. A strong vitality is generally referred to young people when the body can tolerate and recuperate quickly. Low vitality is generally ascribed to older people where less input makes for greater disruption to the body and emotions. Of course, there are older people with great vitality. These people are usually not negatively affected much and often like to spend time with young people. On the other side, there are young people with low physical stamina and or emotionally easily affected. The purpose of homeopathy is to free up the inherent Individual's vitality thereby restoring health.

For most people, outside of medications control over disease is limited to biochemical choices as such diet including supplements, exercise and mental hygiene such as meditation or relaxation, all of which are good choices, and I am naturally a fervent practitioner of them. Environment and stress are substantially more difficult to deal with in everyday life and we generally try to gain some control over them by recruiting the help of many professionals such therapists, medications, etc. Another category that influences our health is our heredity, which we are told we don't have any control over as if is all engraved in stone. It could not be further from the truth. Some genetic information changes very rapidly and some of it doesn't change much. The fact that we have one nose, two ears, one mouth, two arms, two legs, etc., does not change easily, but genes, much like everything else in nature, are not a one dimensional operation. Some genes change all the time, In fact, anything going on in the body involves genes so we can make this general affirmation: we can eventually find a gene for any disorder. The problem is what comes before the gene. What puts genes in motion? Indeed, it is the Vital Force. Without the Vital Force, nothing happens, neither life nor health or disease.

What is new here is that by concentrating on the Vital Force homeopathy bypasses today's biochemical model of disease and goes straight to the source of the problems. The bypass is the key to act directly upon the individual's *dynamis* to return it to a state of health.

The life force keeps us alive and at best it maintains health; it is not capable of curing or lessening or overcoming disease on its own unless it is a self-limited acute illness. If the *dynamis* were capable of doing so there would never have been any need for any type of medicine. At best the life force maintains health, if it doesn't the second best it can do is adapt. This life force can only adapt if the adversity is not lethal. Adaptation leads to evolution or change. Change in turn leads to the nature of Nature: diversity. For the purpose of our short lives, however, diversity does not help us since evolution takes many generations. Take, for example, the antibiotic-resistant microorganisms we have now. It took several generations of microorganism mutation to arrive at that result. As individuals, we don't have that kind of time. Incidentally, homeopaths predicted this antibiotic predicament as soon as antibiotics came out. Once we accept the concept of the Vital Force, it is easy to understand the shortcomings of today's suppressive and manipulative medical thinking. Suppression of symptoms with medication simply becomes the suppression of body processes, which in turn forces the *dynamis* into further mistunement - it strikes me as counterproductive! Although invisible, the Vital Force is as real as gravitation is invisible. The Vital Force and the material body are an indivisible whole in health and otherwise.

Among the most important advantages of the biodynamic approach is the recognition of patterns of diseases belonging to the physical, emotional and mental planes within the context of life. The integration of symptoms seemingly disconnected but in truth interconnected between the different parts of our body and our Being is critical for the homeopath's understanding of the imbalance in the Vital Force. Symptoms are not trivial. They are crucial and purposeful and albeit disagreeable to us, they represent the most perfect reaction of the *dynamis* upon the organism. In fact, all symptoms are organized by the *dynamis* in the organism just like it has organized the body with the liver, the heart, the lungs, with two legs below the torso and a head on top of the neck .

To the homeopath, tissue changes represent the effect of disorder. Once the mistunement of the Vital Force starts, it generally does not stop until the proper dynamic curative agent is brought in to resonate upon the *dynamis* of the disorder. The homeopath's sole concern is the Vital Force expressed through the physical, emotional and mental levels. This is why homeopaths talk about treating the person and not the disease. It cannot be confused that a homeopath treats disease, as he looks at sick people not diseases. Our life force cannot be attacked or infected by anything. An infection is the result, the end result of the impingement upon the Vital Force.

The homeopath seeks to elicit a response of the body's innate *dynamis* by understanding the language of the mistunement of the Vital Force, which can only be told by the person suffering from it. Only the person afflicted can give an account of the condition in him according to the symptoms he complains of and by the alterations in him that are perceptible to his senses. As a homeopath, I understand the only person with all the answers is not myself but rather the one with the ailment. Only the person who can describe his symptoms and the experience of them can truly explain and express what is going on inside of him. The only answer I give at the end of that process is what I think the remedy is. This is difficult to understand because we are so used to relying on technology to tell us how we are. Technology can only tell us how we are on the gross anatomical level such as a tumor, blocked artery and cellular functions are concerned, but it cannot and will not tell anyone how we feel. This is one more departure for homeopathy from the model we are used to. How many people are told they are just fine and yet don't feel well? "I know there is something wrong with me," people say. Many say they have been to the most prominent physicians. Everything has been examined, tested and they say, "You are not sick. You don't have a disease." But as sure as day turns to night, there is a problem, they don't feel right and eventually there will be a disease but only when the damage is so extensive that a label can be put upon it. That is playing catch up to disease.

The beauty of homeopathy is that it not only accepts the way people feel but that feelings are absolutely integrated into the search for the most perfect homeopathic remedy. We simply recognize that the way people feel is part of the way people are affected by illness.

The skill of the homeopath is to recognize and understand the mistunement of the Vital Force through the symptoms told by the person describing them. If the sufferer is well listened to and understood, the homeopath should perceive what needs to be corrected. Attentive listening and precise questioning lead to the proper remedy chosen according to the precise understanding of the disturbed Vital Force represented on the physical, emotional and mental level. The questions always forms a direct line from the main complaint to the deeper level of experience. Each question is designed to lead to the proper remedy, nothing else. As individuals, we ignore the deeper levels of disorder, we are not used to speaking about a disease in a deeper way than to say "something hurts." It is also true that we discount some of our suffering as irrelevant. Or, we may just have gotten so used to suffering that any greater connection seems absurd.

Take, for example, a simple bee sting. Some people may not have much of a reaction at all, physical or otherwise; it is a bee sting that within five minutes will not be felt. Someone else on the other hand might go into a major allergic reaction. Both of these reactions are distinguishingly individual on the physical level only, but there are also people who might be affected emotionally with a deep desire to run seeking help in all directions out of fear of being stung again. Someone else might get very irritated by it and might want to kill the bee at once. Another might be indifferent at the moment only to become belatedly concerned in the evening after seeing the arm still swollen. These are not far-fetched reactions, as I have seen them all and each has required a different homeopathic remedy.

Now imagine all the people suffering from Crohn's disease or Lupus or any other degenerative disease, the different possibilities of experience are almost endless. At the most superficial level all suffer from similar symptoms of their own disease but at the deeper levels of Physical, Emotional and Mental (PEM) it becomes a very individualized matter.

The immediate result of looking at the Vital Force as the total source of suffering is, of course, not only the lifting of the afflictions but overall a healthier individual emotionally and mentally. What is really exciting is that when an individual is truly healthier through the restoration of his or her vitality then the next generation is also healthier because the disordered state is not passed on. Imagine a generation that is less likely to get sick because their parents' *dynamis* is healthier. I just saw a 19-year-old young lady recently who had chronic throat infections mainly treated with repeated courses of antibiotics. Accompanying the throat issues was a difficulty in feeling integrated in a group of friends. She felt as though she should scream in order to be heard but couldn't lest she be further ostracized. With the proper remedy, she is healthier in a fundamental way on all levels (PEM) and it is far less likely that her children will inherit her Vital Force disorder. It is fascinating to me to see that the concept of inheritance or genetic makeup was always part of homeopathy in a very practical way, albeit in a very different way than is commonly thought of today.

Homeopathy is not psychotherapy and nor were the patient's throat problems psychosomatic either. The totality of what she experienced physically, emotionally and mentally about her throat formed a gestalt. Understanding her experience of it all was necessary to recommend the most perfect homeopathic remedy and lift the whole disorder.

In the cases that follow, you will see how it all comes together in the consultation room. You will see how it is all wonderfully logical and rather awe-inspiring. You will understand why homeopathy is made up of two words. *Homeo* meaning "similar" and *pathy* meaning "what one feels."

Every remedy exhibits particular actions, which do not come about in exactly the same way from any other of a different kind.

Samuel Hahnemann

CHAPTER 2

THE LOGIC OF A HOMEOPATHIC REMEDY

As we have seen, the homeopath's first concern is the understanding of the vital disorder as described by the individual in feelings, functions and sensations. Nothing can be done until all the pieces of the puzzle come together clearly in his mind.

Second, the duty of the homeopath is to choose a homeopathic substance to lift of the particular dysfunction. This is what we call "the remedy." It is chosen upon the physical, emotional and mental state as expressed by the affected individual. It is absolutely tailored to the totality of the person's complaints.

The remedy must fit perfectly all aspects of the disorder. The vital disorder cannot be turned into order by something that is antagonistic to it. As I began to explain before, the homeopathic concept is not only in a remedy, it is all around us. Take a "horse whisperer." His approach to tame the horse is to go with the horse. The goal is to acquire a deep understanding of the horse, in return the horse trusts deeply and is willing to form a bond. The end result makes a better team than with the old, submissive, dictatorial but still widely practiced approach. The old approach is to force ourselves upon nature and to submit it to our will. This is in effect what we do when we take a medication. We try to coerce nature - the body in this instance - to act in a specific way.

Our bodies are made up of trillions cells. Millions of cells are born and die each second of our life. As a homeopath, I feel that to interfere with such an awesome process is like jumping into the middle of a stampede and try to divert it in a particular direction. It is impossible! This is analogous to what medicine does currently. In homeopathy we do not oppose the body, but rather use remedies that act like the horse whisperer. When there is gentle accurate force in the right place then no opposing force is needed. The homeopathic remedy acts upon the Vital Force in as gentle of a way as the horse whisperer acts upon the horse because it offers the least resistance against the body and therefore can act deeper and faster than anything else.

Granted it is rather counter-intuitive or unfamiliar for most of us to think this way about what ails us, particularly since the antagonistic allopathic medical system we are familiar with is the only one we know. By virtue of being the only one we know, it is difficult to leave it for something else we don't know. Only with the necessity that ailments place upon us are some of us willing to rethink our common beliefs.

Understanding as in the example of the horse whisperer leads to a state of ease. I understand you, you understand me. There is resonance, it is harmonious and in harmony everything works well. Resonance is the language of music, too; it is highly universal, and it can affect us deeply. A friendship or a relationship work on the principles of resonance, as well. Look at this phrase in *TIME* magazine during the recent presidential campaign: "That a stump speech could have such power and *resonance* came from Edwards' own life (experience) story." We vote according to the message that has the most "resonance" with us. Democracy is based on the concept of resonance. The candidate with the most resonance with the population wins and unless the candidate changes his tune once elected, his message is what the population has chosen as being the best for itself at that particular moment.

So the idea of resonance is not foreign to us at all; we are just not at all accustomed to it when it comes to our health care. We are accustomed to the antagonistic system where disease must be attacked. Surely disorder must be removed but look at the language we use. We go to war with illnesses. It is as if we say to the disease, "Hey, you mess with me, I'll mess with you," or, "We're going to beat it." We look at it as combat, warfare. There is a war on this or that disease. Disease is seen as an entity that is bent on taking someone over. It is deeply ingrained in our consciousness, that's how we speak. I was reading recently about radiation centers around the country the size of football fields with 3-foot thick walls to avoid radiation leakage. Do we really think we are going to ultimately cure cancer this way or is it that the only model we know regards disease as something that needs to be brought into submission? I suspect it's the latter, but since it is all we know that's what we do. We wage war upon disease and I am suggesting that there is another more effective and less harmful system.

The homeopath wants to get rid of disorder where it first develops, on the *dynamis* level not at the cellular level. Understanding is the first step. Giving the most accurate remedy is the other. To be most effective the remedy needs to work directly upon the *dynamis*. If the remedy worked directly on the body:

1. It would not be as effective
2. It would work upon the results of disease only, that is to say only upon the tissue changes
3. It would be suppressive

To restore order directly on the *dynamis*, the remedy needs to be dynamic. It is the resonance of the remedy upon the Vital Force of the disorder that initiates the reversing response to illness. The remedy itself does not heal. Only the influence upon the Vital Force actually heals. Since the remedy acts upon the *dynamis*, there is in fact nothing faster than the proper homeopathic remedy to restore health. When you read the cases that follow, ask yourself whether a medication would help on all the levels these people experienced disorder? I seriously doubt the question will be answered in the positive.

A remedy needs to be dynamic. Making a substance dynamic is the business of the homeopathic pharmacies. There are many homeopathic pharmacies around the world whose job it is only to make homeopathic remedies. Homeopathic pharmacies take a natural substance through a process of dematerialization and into a process of *dynamization*. The process itself of changing a raw substance into a dynamic remedy is really not interesting to explain much as no one is interested in how a conventional medication is made. Suffice to say that in the end the remedy is only a vibration of the original substance. As such, it can act perfectly upon our own *dynamis*, our own vibration of disturbance. We have yet to fully understand what happens during this process of *potentization* but Quantum Physics is shedding some real light on this process.

We have thousands of remedies and we are constantly adding to the list. Only the accurate one must be given in order to have a perfect reaction to lift the whole gestalt of the disorder, otherwise little or nothing happens.

Let's take the example of quinine to see how this process happens. In its raw material form it is commonly prescribed for malaria. The amazing thing is if one were to eat enough quinine as to cause a bit of a poisoning one would develop symptoms similar to the symptoms of malaria. In short, the only reason quinine is effective in the treatment of malaria is its similarity to the effect of the disease. The similarity of the symptoms of the poisoning to the symptoms of malaria is the only reason for its great effectiveness in treatment of that disease; but homeopathy goes one step further. Understanding that *similarity* in the healing concept is only one aspect. The true genius of homeopathy is its ability to take any natural substance and make it into a safe dynamic healing agent that can act in a *synergistic* way rather than a well-used "poison."

The similarity is crucial. It must be a perfect match. It is not easy to find the perfect match within several thousands remedies. This idea of the perfect match has inspired some people to call homeopathic remedies parallels, vibrations, intelligences or images. All of these qualitative terms are correct. Whatever the word one uses, they all need to be accurate in order to have resonance. There has to be resonance in order to act. The greater the similarity, the greater the resonance, the greater the depth of action for lifting the state of disorder and returning to a state of health.

In order to give a remedy accurately we must first find out what are its effects. We need to find out what is its similarity. What are the innate symptoms of the substance. This is what we call a *proving*.

Provings are generally conducted in homeopathic schools around the world, as most students must each year take part in a proving. The first- or second-year students choose to take the remedy which has been prepared by the pharmacy of choice of the proving master. Most of the time it is conducted in a double blind fashion. That is to say that nobody knows what the substance is and no one knows who is taking what. During the proving a temporary imprint occurs, not enough to create harm on the physical, emotional and mental level but enough for the prover to experience. The whole process generally lasts between a few days up to a few months for those who are more sensitive to the substance. This is not a harmful process at all; in fact, one comes out of a proving healthier than one came in. It is really the only way to find out its action - there is no getting around it - but remember that this is no longer a raw substance; the remedy is devoid of all chemical toxicity, it is just a vibration. Nobody is drinking snake poison, okay? There is no other way, there is no theory about anything, we must find out the facts. We don't test anything on rats, dogs or other animals. Once we know what the remedy does it becomes a homeopathic remedy we can then give in the clinical setting.

The point of a proving is to find the core manifestation of the original substance as it translates in the human body. One could say we are looking for its archetype expressing itself morphologically through nature. This is what we call the *essence*. What is the essence of gold, the essence of a spider or the essence of the rose? How do the thorns fit in this symbol of love? How does the essence of the dog fit into the animal that is wild but is totally domesticated? Each substance has an essence. For example when we say, "This person is like an animal," we intuit an essence.

Nowadays we have refined our techniques of case history or "case taking" so much that you will see some people describe the disorder in the very terms as to describe the remedy / substance needed. This is when the meeting point of essence and vital disorder is reached in its innermost core. I have heard a mother describe a cough as a "tinny" cough for which I gave *Stannum*, originally tin. Other symptoms also fit the remedy picture. That meeting point where the patient is in total contact with the archetypal substance in relation to his condition is the ultimate and deepest place for the remedy to provoke a healing reaction. The *resonance* of the remedy upon the disordered Vital Force at that point can only bring health. There is no room for anything else, no vacuum, only the removal of disorder in its most fundamental point. In resonance everything is easy. To arrive at resonance is not simple but its result is worth many, many times the effort. There is no war here, just the annihilation of disorder through resonance. In this context there is no need to attack disease.

So we see that a homeopathic remedy is a substance of a very precise nature acting in perfect resonance with the vital force. The capacity of the remedy to act directly upon the mistunement of the Vital Force is the power and genius of homeopathy.

A word should be said about the consistency of remedies. We are accustomed to hearing about new breakthroughs in medicine virtually every day. Well, our remedies don't change, they are an eternal truth because they are scientifically accurate. We just keep adding new ones. What was true 200 hundred years ago is still accurate today. Remedies don't change because they rest upon solid simple principles heretofore explained. Once one taps into what is *essential* then there is no change because it is truth. It cannot change because it is accurate. It is much like Einstein's theory of relativity. It won't change, we can just understand it better. I mentioned music before. A piece of music is similar in that it is forever. It stands on its own for time immemorial. A remedy is the same, it has its resonance and once discovered it remains forever vibrant, clear and useful. There are pieces of music that stand the test of time and others that go by the way side. Our remedies are the same, as well. Some remedies are used more frequently than others and some are not used as commonly. In my practice, I often recommend remedies that are rather rare because they often offer more specificity and individuality than the more well-known ones. It is like listening to many different pieces of music rather than only the Top 40.

Homeopathic remedies come mainly in two forms, a little white tablet or in a liquid form. They are both the same since the tablet form is rolled in the liquid. It is only a matter of preference on the part of the homeopath. The tablet form is white with a slightly sweetish taste and generally half the size of an apple seed.

At times, I am asked how can this tiny little tablet do so much? Well, it does so for all the reasons explained above. Again, it is a matter of accuracy and resonance. When both of these are present there is no fighting on the inner levels. Little is needed and much can be achieved because at its core Nature wants to thrive, it is always trending positive. The remedy is only a catalyst for change on the Vital Force that permeates the whole organism on the physical, emotional and mental levels. As it permeates everywhere, it forms one whole totality and therefore one remedy is needed. The result of such a process is a very gentle removal of disorder without weakening, causing anguish, ordeal or pain to the patient. Restoring health is not a complicated, sordid or difficult affair according to these principles. It is merely an effortless resonance. We don't purge, we don't ask to make drastic changes in your diet, we don't tell you to stand on your head or force yourself into a program that you would inevitably leave within a few months. At times some old symptoms may come back temporarily, a reversal of the disorder that will lead to long lasting healing. All of it is simply perfect.

When a person falls ill, it is initially only this life force, everywhere present in the organism... mistuned to such abnormality... that it imparts to the organism the adverse sensations and induce in the organism the irregular functions that we call disease.

Samuel Hahnemann

CHAPTER 3

Health is good but...
A HEALTHY STATE IS BETTER!

"I am healthy. I feel great." Though we say that mainly out of courtesy once that veneer is slightly rubbed off it often turns out that the person saying it is either taking several medications, is not feeling happy or is simply avoiding going to the doctor for a chronic condition. The fact is, according to "Partnership to Fight Chronic Disease" (PFCD), 130 million Americans suffer from chronic conditions and according to the CDC seven out of ten deaths are attributable to chronic diseases. Saying and feeling healthy is very different than *being* healthy physically, emotionally and mentally.

We spend an enormous amount of money on disease - two trillion dollars worth and climbing. *Health* is obviously not something many of us are concerned with. We tend to take the approach "if it is not broken, don't fix it," but too many of us take that motto to the grave. Some of us go to the gym - that's a good thing - though too often it is just a faint calorie burning session having more to do with the way we want to look rather than with our physical health let alone the feeling we can indulge in ice cream just because we did fifteen minutes on the treadmill.

There are two basic measures most of us can take to improve our basic health:

1. Cut our daily calorie count by 40%
2. Drink enough water to have fairly clear urine
   (Drinking six to eight glasses a day is actually a pretty good simple advice considering we are mainly made of water.)

With these two steps we can help ourselves live longer and healthier lives yet very few of us do it.

Calorie restriction is the only "diet" that has proven to be life-extending. There are several reasons for that. The primary reason is that if we limit food the body begins to burn its own fat. On a long-term basis this is a far more effective way to improve health than anything else. When the body goes into reverse metabolism, using its own food in the process, it becomes more efficient at using nutrients from food. Fat creates cushions that prevent the proper functioning of organs. Look at marbled steak. You can just imagine how that fat totally impedes with the functioning of the muscle. It is the same throughout our body. Excess fat impedes function, getting rid of it helps.

Something else happens when we eat less food. The body and the mind begin to avail themselves of a different kind of energy. Food energy is but one type of energy but there are several other kinds. Since we are not self-propelled the kind of fuel we use for our body contributes to our health. We need to understand these different kinds of fuels.

When you decide to cut 40% of calories (assuming you are an average American eating about 3000 calories a day), you begin to watch the food you eat more closely. Most people add a lot of green or other sun-ripened food. What happens then is that we become more in tune with the sun plane rather than the earth plane. Think of green foods and fruits as sun foods. This is a higher and more refined energy source than meat. I believe it is one of the reasons why when you go to a poor country most of the time we are quite taken by the local people's kindness, broad smiles and generosity. This is because of the poverty, the food they eat is mostly sun food. By default, it is less expensive; they eat higher energy food. Sun foods also relates to mannose, which are crucial for nutrient utilization from cellular communication.

Whether we recognize it or not, the sun provides us with a supple higher energy we make use of all the time. The condition Seasonal Affective Disorder (SAD), considered to be a depression with apathy, is a direct example. As soon as the longer days of spring come back the condition lifts.

Lastly, as far as food is concerned, there is fasting. For whatever length of time, it is the most profound and radical way to try to tap into that solar energy. I think tapping into this higher energy is the reason why most religions place a big emphasis on fasting.

All this begs the question: If everyone were to do this, would we all be healthy? The answer is simply "No." We would just be a little healthier. Nature would have it that a vital healthy state is far deeper, sophisticated, significant and ultimately more rewarding. If it were as easy as eating salad everyday I think we would all be doing that. These practices help because they create less stress upon the Vital Force but most of them don't go deep enough. Have you ever had the feeling that even though you are doing everything right you are still not feeling well? You are eating right, going to yoga classes, meditating, going to the gym and you are still not feeling 100%. This was exactly the situation in "Gaya, a case of insomnia" in part two of this book.

All of the good advice magazines devote their pages to helping one feel great rarely provide a long-lasting answer. Only the vital state, which is deeper than the PEM can provide a solid ground upon which one can reliably stand to feel 100%. If nutrition is so crucial, and in that sense I loosely join the medical establishment, how can we explain Eskimos eating mostly meat and doing well? Remember that we are mammals. As such, most mammals eat few foods, monkeys have limited diets, whales just eat fish, lions eat meat, etc., and do well. Are we omnivores by opportunity or by nature? My point is that, in the end, nutrition does not explain much and the food debate of high carbohydrate versus low carbohydrate diet and everything in between only adds to the argument. It is not worth joining it for it is not the answer to a perfectly healthy state though it does contribute to good health.

What really grabs our attention is when we don't feel well. At that very moment, our sole preoccupation is to get rid of the pain or dysfunction that afflicts us. Once we have pain we scramble for any plan of action. Anything will do and the medical profession has responded in kind with ever more powerful drugs to eradicate ourselves of our ills. It is simple law of supply and demand. That combined with a philosophy of inevitable escalation has created awesome medications all the way to nuclear medicine. Who would have thought? In a way, since pain and dysfunction is what attracts our attention we should look at them as an opportunity for healing on deeper levels than we are accustomed to.

While it is understandable that someone in pain wants relief, no one is asking where does pain come from? Why do we get pain, discomfort or dysfunction? We know the physiology of it but since life is mainly an experience, can we take our own life experience out of the pain and dysfunction? I don't think so. Since the experience of each individual is perceived differently shouldn't that have something to do with the character of our pains and dysfunctions? I, indeed, wholesomely think so and my profession proves to me that it is correct every day.

Looking at all this entails looking at what I call the *vital state of disorder*. I am not talking about looking at separate parts, but rather looking at the whole disturbance from *one* central and crucial point of solution.

We are part of the Cosmos – we are part of the wholeness of its whole. Indeed, we may think we are insignificant but we are nonetheless part of it and ideally we fit like a piece of a puzzle fits into the rest of it. This may sound like grandiose talk but it is absolutely real. As I spoke of tapping into solar energy, we can also tap into universal energy. As being part of life, part of the universe, can we consider ourselves separate from its energy?

We can ask ourselves: How does a cell emerge? How does the cell incorporate into the coherent system of the universe? How does it become part of it? We are part of the cosmic system and its inter-dependence which in turn is colored by the influences of our solar system. For example it is well known that emergency personnel receive more calls on full moon days than any other during the month. It is also well known there is less crime after an electrical storm, clearing the air of negative accumulated influences.

We are not fragmented individuals. We are one whole with our direct environment, location, family, work, school, country, and universe. I come from the French Alps. That gives me a granite quality that some have difficulty understanding. If I were from a hot, sunny, beach environment I would have different qualities. Living in New York further influences my natal traits. All this colors me as an individual but this is not what we are interested in. Homeopathy does not interest itself in these aspects but rather in the experience of the disordered Vital Force. That does not change by a different locale or time or social status. We are all equal in suffering and disorder. It may be described in a different way but at the vital, more universal level it is expressed the same way and the pain is the same.

A Healthy State is an *authentic* state as is schematically represented in Figure 1. There is one wholesome individual capable of adapting to circumstances without being adversely affected by them. That state can adapt widely to strong stresses. The stronger the Vital Force the more it can sway and adapt freely. In that vital healthy state nothing clouds or interferes with the physical, emotional or mental levels. All functions work in perfect synergy with each other for the higher purposes of one's life.

Being in a healthy state does not mean life is perfect. It does mean that we are in perfect synergy within ourselves on the PEM and the rest of the world. The wholesomeness within one's inner self, our family, our friends, our community, the world and the universe is the issue. It is synergy that makes life easier, not external acquirable or non-acquirable factors.

As such, it is the sole interest of homeopathy to return individuals as close to that state as possible. The homeopath is only interested in removing the internal alteration of the *life principle* (Vital Force) and consequently the totality of the disorder, only then is health restored, at the level of the Vital Force on the Universal plane.

A strong Vital Force is the exact opposite of rigid. It means it is the most adaptable. Life presents us with many difficult situations in the form of physical ailments, emotional challenges and mental stresses. Our ability to deal with them without harm is determined by the strength or weakness of our Vital Force. The strength of the Vital Force lies in its ability to "roll with the punches" without attachments. Depending on its strength, situations begin to affect us. We react to these situations in patterns after which a groove or tendency begins to form according to the limitations of our Vital Force and the path of least resistance within our body. This is the path of disorder that eventually as a last resort, begins to manifest as disease.

Sometimes, the path of disorder feels separate. This is when people say, "I don't feel like myself." In most chronic disorders, as our feeble Vital Force looses its ground, it becomes difficult to distinguish it from ourselves. Little by little the groove becomes a seemingly undivided part of us seeping deeper and deeper affecting us on the PEM levels. We can even come to perceive it as part of our personality. It is not who we are but it definitely permeates and affect us. For example, someone who gets angry easily is affected by a disordered Vital Force on the emotional level. I once saw a testimony by Mr. Rogers of the television program "Mister Roger's Neighborhood" before Congress. His statement was a textbook perfection of calmness in the face of great opposition. I recommend everyone watch it on Youtube.com. He demonstrates the healthy emotional state of calmness. His show was very much about developing a healthy emotional state in children. As such, he had a very accurate view of the expression of a healthy emotional state.

Some people can handle enormous stresses with little effort. Others are "sensitive," that is to say not as healthy as they could be and can only handle very little. On the physical level, a simple example might be people who get colds easily. As soon as the first cold day hits they catch a cold. For others, it could be 20°F below zero and they don't get sick. Conversely, some people can handle great stresses in their relationships and others are frazzled as soon as the husband is not home by 7:30 PM. Homeopathy restores harmony within by strengthening the Vital Force dramatically increasing the likelihood of living with better health.

Figure 1 is a simple sphere representing wholeness. It can be further improved by incorporating the PEM levels. Schematically this can be shown as three areas shading into each other. It is not possible to compartmentalize the three levels because they intermingle within the entire organism.

Emotions reside in the physical and the physical resides in the emotional. Candace Pert, Ph.D., scientific director of Rapid Pharmaceuticals, Inc., coined the term, "molecules of emotions." As she demonstrates some of these molecules can now be measured in the physical body, which I prefer to call that the physicality of emotion. What homeopathy interests itself with is actually beyond molecules. To say there are molecules of emotions is riveting, of course, but it is like saying the Big Bang is the beginning of the Universe. OK, that may be correct but what was there before the Big Bang. We need to look beyond the physical. To look only in the physical world for our health is like physics not looking beyond the material world.

The Vital Force comes before the body. That is the level of Authenticity. That level is not a one dimensional, physical mechanism. It is a fluid process with one level influencing the other, much like an interminable dance of one thing influencing the other. The key to find an accurate homeopathic remedy with perfect resonance upon the disorder is to understand the disorder at this universal level. This is demonstrated at length throughout the cases I present and their discussion. The fact that we are not accustomed to looking at this intermingling as a logical, organized, interdependent unit of PEM with its root in the universe and that so much gets lost in translation in-between the levels or even gets ignored does not mean it doesn't exist.

In a vital state of disorder, the exciting cause or the physical trigger to a large extent is only the beginning. What matters is the reaction or the pattern of the disorder affecting the person. In autism, for example, many people concern themselves with the mercury or Thymerisol in the vaccines. This is fine, some children have fared well taking the mercury detoxification route. This is the rationalist, linear, one-dimensional and physical school of thought of which modern medicine adheres to. It is an ever more sophisticated route of cause and effect. This route has the unfortunate effect of providing an argument to the people opposed to the theory; in this particular case that mercury has anything to do with autism. They simply point out that if it were so then all children should be afflicted and chelating it from the body should be successful all the time.

Homeopathy concerns itself with the demonstration of the affectation. In the previous example, the reaction to the poison on the PEM is what is important. Mercury is not the disorder but rather only a part of it, the reaction of the mind and body to it is more important as that state is more encompassing of the whole of human nature and, therefore, more accurate. This is why there is limited success with taking the route of removing (chelating) the mercury out of children with autism spectrum disorder (ASD). The disorder does not change according to external influences but they can determine the degree of severity upon the Vital Force.

Homeopathy acts from the very center of disorder, rather than through a theory, so these arguments are totally avoided. Understanding the pattern of affliction leads to the remedy capable of reaching deeper into the vital level and removal of the disorder.

Authenticity, on the physical level means to be free of any disturbance of pain, malfunction or discomfort. One does not need to be an athlete to be healthy, though exercise is naturally important. Walking and contemplating are two important functions for the health of the human body. I remember reading about Mother Teresa's mission in Calcutta. She made sure the sisters were living away from the mission itself and Mother Teresa insisted that they walk to it. The purpose was that they would get exercise, they'd be able to chat, laugh, giggle and disconnect from their work. Naturally, Mother Teresa had an understanding of what contributes not only to good health but also to a healthy state. Contemplation doesn't have to be very sophisticated; it can be as simple as being curious about things that cross our lives every day.

In homeopathy, what we are further interested in is the integration of the PEM. In the example of Sandra's case of sinusitis she says, "*It* takes all my attention." This is an example of physical dysfunction (sinusitis) overlapping into the emotional level, "it takes all my attention." Knowing that "*it* takes all my attention" is measurably interesting and once we find out that "*it*" is also perceived as having prevented her from having a career in show business, professions that are usually tracked by the spotlight and attention, then it becomes fascinating. Our actions correspond exactly to what our clouded mind/emotion perceive as happening to us. To the homeopath, that perception combined with the physical state is essential to understand the deeper vital state to choose the appropriate remedy.

In a state of physical health there is no PMS during your menstrual cycle, no physical restrictions or pain or any dysfunction in the body such as brain, heart, kidneys, gastro-intestinal etc. Any deviation from that and one is experiencing disorder.

The emotional level can be a fragile one, indeed. It is the bridge between the physical and the mental. As such, it has vulnerabilities. I like to compare it to the knee in the body. Its function as a bridge makes it quite prominent in the functioning of an individual and so the emotional state of health is prominently displayed. When someone enjoys a healthy emotional state there is no anger, anxiety or panic at external stimuli. There is no fear or phobias even about health or death. One does not suffer from anguish, fears or feeling of a lower nature such as jealousy. There is no laziness or apathy. Dissatisfaction, revenge, irritability or sadness does not see the light of day. None of these are present; there is only gorgeous harmony within and without. Take a person who is being nice when he is sick. Is the niceness because he is nice by nature or nice because of a fear of being alone while he is sick? In the first instance niceness does not have anything to do with the disorder. In the second it can be used to understand the deeper part of the disorder.

When the mental level is functioning without impediment, the memory is great and the intellectual faculties are keen and clear. With a lack of clarity in thought and expression one's thinking becomes disturbed. One is not absent-minded and there is no lack of concentration. There is no lethargy or dullness. Logic is sharp with rationality, coherence and logical sequence, without any room for mental confusion. Destructive delirium or paranoid ideas are totally absent as are delusions. There is creative service for the good of others as well as for the good of oneself. The question is not can I be smarter but rather can I be clearer?

The disorder of the VF should not be confused with the personality or character of an individual though it seeps through to affect the personality. For example, on the mental level, the level of intelligence has to do with the person. One does not have to be the most intelligent person in the bunch to be the most mentally stable. In fact...! The mental level is the most crucial to humanity. It is our mental acuity that has gotten us here and not our ability to dig a hole. Stephen Hawking is arguably the most brilliant physicist of our time though he is wheelchair bound with amyotropic lateral sclerosis and can't even speak; yet, he has contributed enormously to our understanding of the universe. The world is replete with people who because of their clarity of mind help people without even knowing it.

Figure 1.

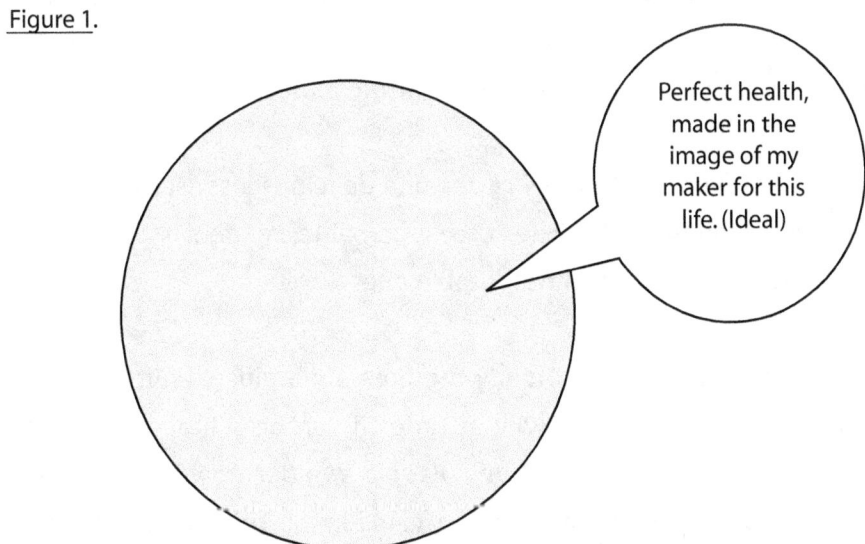

Perfect health, made in the image of my maker for this life. (Ideal)

To understand the disorder at the vital level, the homeopath needs to bring it alive. After all, we are interested in Life more than anything else and how the disorder affects or interferes with it. "It," the disorder, is not static, "it" has life and is part of life. Today's skill of the homeopath is to bring "It" to life by bringing the person to describe it in such fine internal details that it is easy to determine what the remedy is. Case taking becomes a slow "impersonation" of the disorder. Disorder is an experience. The homeopath seeks to involve the person in describing the disorder as he/she experiences it. The expression at that level is what the homeopath needs to understand in order to accurately recommend a remedy.

Each disordered state is to be identified into a remedy state. This is all very dynamic and full of life. This is done through the expression of the disorder alone. The Life Force is only discernible by manifestations of the disorder in feelings and functions.

"The body is a material instrument for life, it is not conceivable without the life imparted to it by the instinctual, feeling and regulating *dynamis*, just as the life force is not conceivable without the organism. Consequently, the two of them constitute a unity." *Hahnemann*

When one works with it every day one develops a sense of it. At the level of Authenticity, the Life Force is palpable. You feel it just like you feel love or any other immeasurable energy.

Finding the restorative remedy requires a merging of left and right brain functions, which is why at times it can be a little difficult for people to answer my questions. People wonder how my questions have anything to do with what they came in for. The questioning is so different that it even raises doubt in their mind. When I ask, "What is the feeling?" many people don't know how to answer. When people can no longer answer the questions I often describe what I am looking to understand with a drawing as in Figure 1: You, in perfect health. Then I explain that the disturbance, as in Figure 4, is very unique to you. It forces the Vital Force to cope and what I need to understand is the *true* expression of the Vital Force, lying deeper than the PEM handling the disharmony.

The homeopath is only interested in restoring a healthy vital state by removing the disorder upon the VF as is schematically represented in Figure 2. We do not seek to cure but rather remove disorder.

Is the removal of the appendix a cure? Is the removal of uterine fibroids a cure? The ample cases in Part 2 make perfectly clear that to the homeopath the disappearance of ills is an indirect one. How else could a substance into which nothing physical is left act upon the removal of a malady? Indeed, it seems impossible. What is possible is demonstrated here. The disappearance of an ailment is a dynamic one. Cure may be the removal of symptom but what I am interested in is erasing the disordered state and restoring freedom to the individual on the PEM. Figure 2 also shows the disorder seeping and interfering with the person. The depth of the encroachment depends on the "seepage" of the disorder into the person. Little-by-little, this encroachment brings a lack of freedom upon the person all the way to being terminal; it does not stop until we die unless we are given the proper homeopathic remedy. It is a like a river cutting its way through the mountains and the valleys. We can only hope that our own river is more like a stream rather than the Colorado through the Grand Canyon.

A return to true health is a return to Authenticity. It is the uncovering of the core as it was meant to be by the Highest Graces at this point in time of our lives. It is really the level we instinctively want to achieve. How the three levels (PEM) interact and influence each other has much to do with our Vital Heredity as you can see in the children's cases. Most of them reflect what I think is the most forgotten aspect of homeopathy, which is the improvement of health from one generation to the next at the deepest level.

Figure 2.

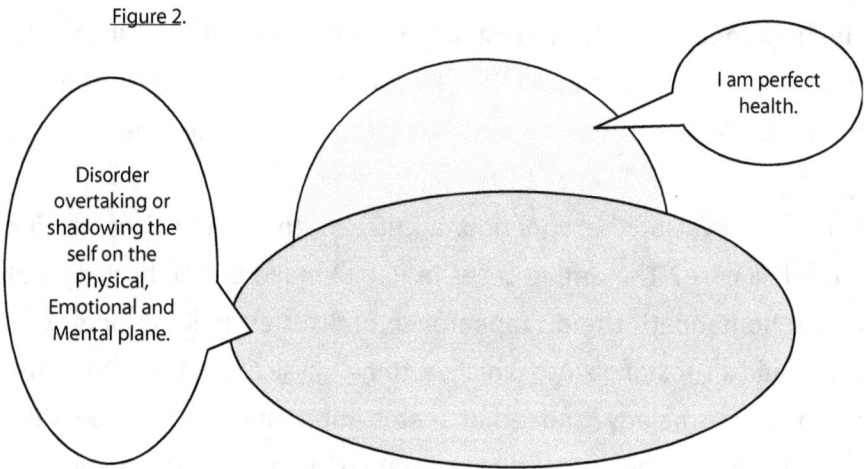

Whether someone has a lot of emotional issues but few physical and deep issues on the mental level depends upon the path of least resistance within the person's constitution. The better the constitution of the parents the more chances the children will benefit from great health. The shaded area is what the homeopath is interested in. The goal of the homeopath is to peel that back so that only your whole Self remains.

In Figure 3, the shaded area peeling back represents the disorder. However, it is more accurate to look at the disorder as fading out. The homeopathic remedy does not cut or suppress symptoms but rather strengthens the healthy Vital Force by overcoming the forces impinging upon it. All of this process takes place as a *dynamic* power acting from the deepest level within outward. Nothing is missed, from the deepest outwardly to the most superficial, from the most vital to the least vital retracing to a healthier time by the action of the remedy upon it, reconnecting to that time and state of Authenticity.

Figure 3.

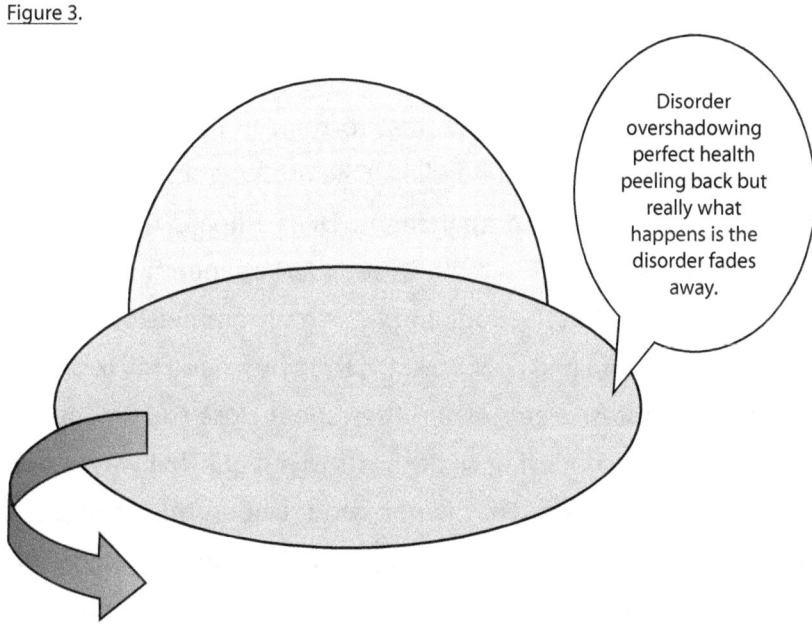

Disorder overshadowing perfect health peeling back but really what happens is the disorder fades away.

A great state of health on the PEM is rare. In my whole life, I have met only one such person I will call Jack. I remember a friend of mine speaking about him. He made this comment to me: "It seems that even if a volcano were to erupt right next to him, he would be fine." What do you mean? I asked. He answered, "He is so grounded, you get the sense that he would not panic. He would be fine, keep himself functioning optimally and do what needs to be done only because he will not be affected by it." I loved it. He had essentially described a harmonious state of emotion.

This person's body was morphologically strong kind of like Charlston Heston in *Ben Hur* without pumping iron. He felt strong in it but without showing strength. He ate well but not fanatically. His intellect was very keen and creative. It is rare to have all three.

This individual was working on oil rigs in Alaska. Then he went on vacation to France and after visiting museums decided to become a sculptor. He did, by getting a Master's degree. He then moved to the Dominican Republic where he now lives.

Here is another example in contrast to that. I once lived for a few weeks in a seedy apartment building. One morning someone planted a fire bomb in front of an apartment. Once I heard the noise and commotion outside I took a look. As soon as I opened the door black smoke poured in. I shut the door and woke my roommate up. I was not terribly worried but I had concerns. On the other hand my roommate took fifteen minutes to get up and then spent close to 10 minutes in front of his closet wondering what shorts to put on. That was lethargy combined with dullness. That is not good. During this same event, the people who were thinking of jumping or screaming in panic were not healthy either, and some, in their panic, got seriously burned.

Since you have come this far into the book, I have the pleasure to announce to you that you probably now understand something about Quantum Theory. Here is an excerpt from "The Leonard Lopate Show" on WNYC, June 17, 2007 discussing teleportation with Michio Kaku, professor of theoretical physics at the graduate center of the City University of New York and co-founder of Field Theory. I happened to listen to it the same day I finished this chapter. My jaw dropped as he mentioned several points I make in these chapters so I suggest applying his insights to homeopathy.

The parts I find important from a homeopathic point of view are underlined.

"Everything vibrates around us (1). We know that from the Quantum theory. If you have two electrons that vibrate in unison, that's called coherence (2). If you then separate these two electrons, an invisible umbilical cord connects these two electrons by vibrating in unison, such that if you jiggle one the other one knows somehow that its partner is being jiggled (3). Now Einstein didn't like this but, hey, we measure this in laboratories every day. Einstein was wrong. So this is how we get two objects linked together by an invisible umbilical cord. And when we have Captain Kirk ("Star Trek") in the future we will have to destroy him in order to create another Captain Kirk on the other side of the room. This creates a problem because the *other* Captain Kirk has all the memories, all the information, all the genetic neural circuits of the original Captain Kirk. And we just saw the original captain being destroyed. But here is another imposter with exactly the same memory DNA genes claiming that he's *the* Captain Kirk. So you kind of wonder where did the soul go (4) when you teleport his atoms."

It is kind of like cloning only it is not like cloning?

"Yes, we're not talking about cloning a child who is a genetic equivalent to you. We're talking about creating you. You that has every single atom the same as you, who claims to be you, but it's not you."

When Professor Kaku says:
1. "Everything vibrates around us" he is affirming that everything around us and within us is *dynamic.*

2. "Vibrate in unison, that's called coherence" seems to me to be a perfect example of one similar affecting another similar which is the basic idea of homeopathy.

3. "An invisible umbilical cord" is what I believe to be the realm of the Vital Force. And when he says that "if you jiggle one, the other one knows somehow that its partner is being jiggled," he is again making the case of homeopathy. One similar substance, the homeopathic remedy, acting upon another similar substance, impacting the disordered Vital Force of an individual.

4. "You kind of wonder where did the soul go?" it goes straight to what I explained in Chapter 1. The Vital Force is not the soul but rather only a conduit for it. Needless to say, I was elated when I heard this explained in such a coherent, beautifully illustrative manner.

As I mentioned in the foreword, homeopathy has always stood on its cases. Now, it is beginning to be understood. This is real and very beautiful.

Enjoy the cases.

Disclaimer:

All comments in the discussion part of the case are meant as illustrations of the homeopathic approach, depth and wholistic nature as well as a tool to point out the differences with medicine.

All cases are edited for brevity and relevancy. I have purposely omitted to include the potency of each remedy given except in one instance where it was important. The potency is often a distraction from the overarching pertinence of finding the correct remedy.

No information contained herein should be construed as medical information or advice.

PART II

The natural healing force within each one of us is the greatest force in getting well.

Hippocrates

JOSEPH

(Early 20's)

MC: ACNE

- Sinusitis
- Mouth sores

Pierre: Please tell me what brings you here?

"Two days ago my sinuses got a lot worse. I feel a pressure at the root of my nose and it seems like there is some swelling at night inside my nose. Everything becomes a lot worse when I lie down on my back. I also get this sensation of closing and opening of my throat. Oddly enough, it gets better if I breathe cold air rather than hot dry indoor air."

Describe the symptoms a little more for me, please.

"Like I said, it is much worse when I lie down on my back. Last week the mucus was clear. One month ago the pressure in my nose kept waking me up. Now my nose stuffs up and then I feel quite irritated by it. There is no doubt that certain foods aggravate the whole thing. It is much worse when I eat creamy, buttery types of foods. I used to drink a lot of milk and I have been told I should cut it down now and I did but I would like to drink more. "

DISCUSSION

Acne is particularly severe on Joseph's upper back with pimples covering the whole area.

I have to admit that up to a few years ago skin conditions were always a challenge for me. For some reason I just was not getting good results. I even turned people with skin problems down. I don't know why it was so because as you can see cases are always taken the same way. I just kept a small trickle of people and then my results started to change, something cleared in my head and now I have the same results as with any other cases. I still like autoimmune cases more; perhaps it is their complexity that appeals to me. I once heard Isaac Bergman say that a simple piece of music can be harder to play than a difficult one. This is very much the way it was for me with these cases.

Acne in this case was the main complaint but because the sinuses were acting up at the time, it was first on his mind. This is a nice, simple example of hierarchy in the body. The sub-acute condition temporarily diminishes the chronic condition. If all things were linear or equal as in the Western medical model this would not happen.

How much milk would you drink, is it a strong craving?

"Well, I really have a strong desire for it, I drink over half a gallon a day. Cutting down on drinking milk has not helped the sinusitis that much. There is one other thing. If I don't eat I get very shaky and irritated."

You said you feel irritated when you don't eat, what do you mean? Could you describe the feeling, please?

"I am quite sensitive about a lot of things I eat. I don't like a lot of things. I have very basic needs in food and I keep it simple. I am also emotionally quite sensitive. I try to be careful and considerate but irritability certainly gets in the way."

How long has the craving for milk been going on, please?

"For as long as I can remember. I had a good childhood but my family is not very close. Since going to college I haven't had much contact with my family. My mother was mildly abusive, I got away from it all and I feel cut off from my family. The problems with my mother did not help; I thought she was being very unfair towards me. I should tell you that I am worried about being hurt. At times, I do feel like I am being hurt for no good reason. I always feel like I have to do a lot for everyone. Perhaps because of that I get sick often. Sometimes I am sick for a full two weeks."

The question then becomes why is the acne regressing when the sinuses are worse? The answer is that there is an order in the body regulated by the vital force. If disease were truly only a physical matter then such an instance would not happen. But disease is a result of the disorder at the level of the vital force hence when the vital force is expressing an acute or sub-acute condition the chronic is overtaken. When people suffer from different conditions at the same time then all of them are co-mingling on a similar level, which is why one remedy is needed for all the conditions at once — they are all part of the general disorder.

This case is a perfect triangulation of sub-acute/chronic issues and parenting problems. In life all three are dealt at different levels. The acute sinusitis is dealt with an OTC drug. A dermatologist treats the acne. The issue with the parents, notably the mother in this case, is dealt with psychotherapy. With the homeopathic approach, which is the reason why I often use such words as "the beauty of homeopathy" or "the genius of homeopathy" is that the whole "triad" can be dealt with deeply and effectively at once. One cannot only turn to psychotherapy to work this whole thing out; the follow-ups are proof of

REMEDY:

Lac defloratum

FOLLOW UP: (6 weeks later)

Pierre: Tell me how you are feeling, please.

"I have been feeling a lot better. The acne is definitely clearing up, that is incredible because I've had it for so long. The fungus on the feet is also better but the soles of my feet have become rough. I don't feel as angry as before. I am more like disgruntled at this moment. I don't feel as reactive as I was prior to taking the remedy. Not getting hurt has always been an ongoing process for me. For some reason, I was thinking about my mother last week and I feel more forgiving towards her. I don't know why that is but I don't have the same feeling about the whole thing as I did before. There is something else I don't know. I don't have the craving for milk like I used to have. "

OK, what about the sinusitis?

"The dryness in the nose is completely gone. I am sleeping well, I can't even remember the last time I had a good night sleep before taking the remedy, it had not happened in such a long time. At this moment it is all a fraction of what it used to be. I do feel like my nose is a little bit dirty. I blow my nose quite a bit but it seems more like an elimination rather than an accumulation. I have not had any mouth sores."

REMEDY:

Continue

that in this case as well as in many other cases presented in this book. It doesn't mean one should not seek to improve oneself further with the help of a professional but if the baseline is much as in Erika's or James' cases (see cases) then decisions are made from a clear, rational mind rather than a cluttered, encroached one.

Lac means milk. In this case the strong craving for milk led me to think that the remedy needed was one of our many milk remedies.
Of course, there were other criteria that dictated the recommendation of a milk remedy.

In the first follow up he talks about the acne and the family situation but not about the sinusitis. In other words, the hierarchy has been re-established and the whole sub-acute condition is beginning to lift. Since it was prominent in the case I ask about it next.

The issue of the craving for milk is the same as in Danna's case (see case) where the craving diminishes dramatically after taking the proper remedy. When health returns, the craving diminishes and becomes more in line with the rest of the body as well. The craving is part of the disorder; it is logical that it should diminish with the removal of the disorder.

GEORGE
(6 yr old)

MC: ADHD
(Attention Deficit Hyperactivity Disorder)

• History of ear infections

Pierre: What can you tell me about your son, please?

Mother: "My son needs consciousness, he is not here. He is super fast in math and he loves to read but he has difficulties staying on tasks and following directions. He has enormous difficulties cooperating."

How does that translate in every day life?

"He hangs out in the bathroom in school and curses at his baby sitter. He walks around a lot, he reads and is great at math."

Please tell me more about Sam.

"He is not very good at making friends in school because he always has his own agenda. Kids don't want to spend time with him. He is a loner. He always seems to be hot. In the middle of the winter he goes out in shorts and a T-shirt and it doesn't affect him at all."

Sam, can you please tell me about your dreams?

Sam: "I'm on a boat, the whole family gets off the boat and I go home but my parents are

DISCUSSION

I present this case because the child is so "out there" and the mother is so fantastic. From the time the child walks in the consultation room he totally avoids me. He might not even have seen me even though I shook his hand. When his mother asks him a question he does not acknowledge her whatsoever. In a strange way it is like "he is not here."

Observation: He has a cracked, red lower lip.

I understand a lot of parents would be happy to see their ADHD kid read and do math. This case is a little bit more than ADHD.

When I tried to get his attention I was met by an absolute inability to focus any kind of attention on me. I repeated his name several times. As I mentioned before it was as

not home. I am totally alone. I pound on the door, I see that it is not locked so I go in and I watch TV. When it's almost time to go to bed a T-rex crashes through the ceiling. A helicopter chases me; it is trying to kill me with water. The T. rex swats the helicopter and saves me. We then go to sleep together."

What kind of food do you like?

Sam: "I like meat and sour stuff."
Mother: "I should tell you he eats like three people and yet he does not gain weight."

Please tell me about the pregnancy.

Mother: "When I first got pregnant I was frenzied for a few of days and then it settled down. The last four months of the pregnancy were very grueling. I had to go on a diet because I was diagnosed with diabetes. I lost 10 lbs during the pregnancy. I was constantly on the go. I was very upset I had to limit what I could eat and I felt tired all the time. Physically, it was draining to be pregnant but the most challenging was the limitations of food. I felt like I was all alone on an island, totally by myself. I can see the city over there but the ferry is not going to come for a long time. It is a desolate place. The ferry has its own agenda."

For my purpose, this is beautiful information. Please continue.

"The ferry is very much like guards in a prison. I am totally at the ferry's mercy and it is absolutely awful."

if he were not here. Nothing registered. In my experience the best way to get children's attention is to ask them about their dreams but in his case he did not even react to that. I insisted and finally he came out of his blankness.

I could not get any more information than that, he didn't want to describe anything to me. He kind of went blank again.

His mother says "He eats like three people" and he was actually underweight. That combined with his insensibility to cold weather were two characteristics that gave me indications for a remedy.

For further information I asked the mother about the pregnancy.

As I am listening to the mother tell her story about having to "limit what she could eat" I am remembering the child's ravenous appetite. She also describes her state wonderfully well.

The mother's unique and eloquently explained state during pregnancy was key. She felt like on an island at the mercy of the ferry.

REMEDY:

Natrum Iodatum 30C

Let me share the *Materia Medica* of Jan Scholten with you. (Dictionary where the remedies are listed and detailed)

"They are completely alone in their struggle for life. It may be a matter of getting something to eat. The most basic right of food is taken away, as well as other rights, such as freedom of movement, freedom of expression and the right to have some belongings. Such a person has no say in the situation and is dependent on the whims of his guard. A third variation is the feeling that all possibilities of escape have been taken away. This is a concentration camp situation."

This description fits Sam most perfectly.

FOLLOW UP:

Pierre: How is Sam?

"His teacher asked me what we did because she has seen a major behavioral improvement in school. When he first took the remedy there was a big improvement in attitude and behavior. Whereas he did not have any signs of conscience before, now it is much better. Like I said, the teacher also noticed the change in behavior and attitude. He does not stay angry as long. He is more eager to please. He is doing more things on his own. Doing his homework is not as nearly as difficult as before because he is not as distracted."

1: It is very difficult to escape from an island, which is why the most famous jails are built there.

2: She felt at the mercy of the ferry much like at the mercy of the guards in a camp. The ferry was withholding the food. She couldn't say anything. She felt her freedom was terribly restricted. The dream of the child reflects the idea of being alone and not being able to escape. The helicopter is right above. One can never escape the searchlight of a helicopter. The child's dream is updated to his time but it is the same state as the mother's during the pregnancy. If we take the child's dream we can't arrive at the remedy unless we ask a lot more questions but once we have the mother's state it makes prefect sense.

This case was the case that started my journey of breakthroughs for the treatment of autism. All of them explained in my upcoming book on autism.

I am very happy to hear that. Can you tell me more?

"He seems to be happier at home. He is not as angry when he wakes up. He is more selective about things he is carrying in his pockets. He used to carry all kinds of little toys in his pockets now when I do the laundry I don't find as many. He used to nudge and gravitate around his brother, now he seems to be more independent."

REMEDY:
Wait

PHONE: (2 weeks later)

Pierre: How can I help you?

"He is coughing, sneezing, and he has a sore throat. He has a bit of a fever."

Is he doing anything out of the ordinary?

"I noticed that he is only asking for cold food or cold O.J. He does not want anything hot or even warm."

REMEDY:

Phytolacca

PHONE: (3 days later)
Pierre: How is Sam?

"I can't believe it. His throat stopped hurting before we arrived at doctor's office so he did not even see him."

The child appears much calmer and somehow in this short amount of time he seems more mature. He said "Hi" to me and looked at me when he shook my hand. He is playing with a toy but he is also paying attention to what his mother is telling me.

With such a good follow up there is no need to give anything at this point. He continues to improve; the Vital Force (VF) is still working its way into better health. The only two times we need to repeat a remedy is when the person stops improving or if there is regression. Eventually the resonance is strong enough for the VF to stay healthy for a long time.

Desiring cold food or drinks during a cold/sore throat is a strange, rare and peculiar (SRP). I should point out that it is unusual for a parent to be aware of such details but his mother is very much in tune. In George's case the mother makes the observation that "before homeopathy I never paid attention to these things."
Here, this mother is very tuned in to this sort of thing.

PHONE: (One week later)

"I can see he is slipping back into his old ways."

REMEDY:

Repeat the constitutional remedy

FOLLOW UP: (Six months later)

How has Sam been lately?

"He is really well. He has been very helpful at home. He is like a different kid. His brother bothers him but he does not respond like before. There is a major difference."

REMEDY:

Wait

FOLLOW UP: (two years later.)

"He has been doing very well in school. He is pleasant. Nowhere near the way he was when I first brought him."

Today, instead of giving an acute remedy like I did I would recommend a repetition of the constitutional remedy. Doing so would probably have avoided the "slipping back" and it would have *dynamized* or strengthened the Vital Force.

Close to two years later he continues to do very well. Now imagine what kind of an adult George would become without a homeopathic remedy. Now a whole new future is opened to him.

MOLLIE
(Early 50's)

DISCUSSION

MC: ANXIETY ATTACKS
- Bursitis in the right shoulder
- Infection in the gums
- Pain along the shin

Pierre: What brings you here?

"I have very bad anxiety attacks. I've always had anxieties but now they've gone through the roof. Since our tragedy I have had to restart the business by myself but I am still in disbelief. It is still a little bit like a dream. We have enormous financial problems and I despair about them. I also have physical problems, which I think are somehow related to this whole situation. I have developed bursitis in the right shoulder, and an infection in the gums. I can't really relax and concentrate because I am very worried. I think I have a lot of anger and I can't get it out or it comes out in strange ways. I am angry with my husband, emotionally I don't trust him, I think he is reckless and I feel kind of bullied by him. I am struggling because I can't be me. I don't know who I am anymore. I have a contradiction: I am easily bullied, and yet I have a strong intuition. I feel like I am in a complete state of imbalance, anxiety and fear. I can't keep any equilibrium; anything can diminish my self-esteem. I feel all out of whack, I have a very

Mollie has a voice like the singer Mary Gray, which sounds slightly like inhaling helium.

Words like "anger" or "can't concentrate" are very broad and convey very little to me. We need to go far deeper in order to perceive the true individual qualities of the disorder. Read on.

heavy heart and I don't feel in harmony with anybody."

Please tell me about being "all out of whack," or not keeping "any equilibrium."

"I have pain up my shin from my ankle to the knee. It is like a hairline up my shin that is quivering. It is not a strong line, it is as thin as a hair yet there is some strength there but it is not consistent."

Could you tell me more about not feeling balanced, please?

"I am an artist; much of my work is about centeredness and non-centeredness. The more you try to go to the center, the more off-centered it becomes. I work with mirrors and glass. It's like seeing yourself and not really seeing you. I work with mirrors, but I diffuse the mirror with netting, so you can't see yourself completely or clearly. Seeing or not seeing clearly is the main idea. It is a fine line, being fragile in parts has been important. I used to listen to Miles Davis to understand that frame of mind. I feel blocked and my own mind is holding me back."

Could you describe feeling blocked, please?

"I have had many tragedies in my life. One of my comforts is anger but then I feel guilty from being angry. I can't really see, or be, I can't open up, and I lose the connection with me, that's if I ever really had it. I am not able to

I ask about feeling "all out of whack" and she answers "I have pain in my shin." The answer to this question is rather off subject. It is very common for people to not answer the questions I ask. In fact, that is the main reason for spending as much time in consultation as we do. Each case presented here is edited down to the most essential for that very same reason.

When she says "It is a fine line," It reminds me of the hairline pain on the shin. Most of the time this kind of serendipity gets lost in the translation between the physical and emotional, my job is to be alert to these un-seeming connections to find them and unwind them down to the root.

In the last answer from a homeopathic point of view she gives a lot of useful information. To keep the flow, I just pick up on the last thing she said.

breathe. It's like a simmering pot inside, like I am inside a cardboard or an armor. It's kind of safe, it's like a black shield. Like a cocoon, not uncomfortable, just limiting or isolating, I am a people person, I like to connect, but people don't connect with me and that causes me great pain and anxiety."

Describe the feeling of being in a cocoon a little more please.

"There is no happiness or sadness, it just is. There are no emotions attached to it, it is kind of the way I feel about life. It is a little nervous in that cocoon. At the time of our tragedy my mind said, "That's that." I was in that cocoon. That has really perplexed me. I had that armor around me, I put a coat over my head until we got back to NY. I could not see or hear anybody. I was in a cocoon. Being in there is like staring without seeing; I can stare for a long time. You lose a certain connection. It is like there is a little bit of a hum, it does not change in frequency or volume, it is a little bit like being dead. It is not unpleasant, it just is. Then I grew concerned about my husband and I had to face everything."

The cocoon is becoming a major theme. The translation of the theme of seeing and not seeing in her art is indeed a reflection of her deeper feeling. In her case it is similar to being in a cocoon, which is a fine line between being and not being or staring and not seeing. The expression of the Vital Force (VF) is all encompassing as in a whole interconnected web. Everything makes sense nothing is lost in translation.

Describe the feeling of losing a certain connection.

"When it comes down to it, I am not sure who I really am. Losing connection is losing connection to my own construct, I am fragile. I am impulsive and from intuition I feel good, but if I have even one question then I become doubtful. For example, a doctor gave me your number. I instinctively called you, but had my husband questioned me before, I would easily have doubted myself. I am not vocal, I hold on to my ideas instead of expressing them. I try not to make waves. When someone calls me then I get very insecure. My job growing up was to take care of everybody. In the cocoon there is groundedness. Some mornings I wake up and I feel grounded, solid and not fragile. Other mornings I am completely fragile. It can go either way but I've always had the thing about breathing. In yoga class I get all anxious and I can't breathe."

It is common to force behavior prematurely onto kids as it is the case here. She had to take care of everybody. Invariably that leads to emotional problems later on in life as if that part of life had not been lived. In this case, she assumed the responsibility of taking care of things but it was not emotionally dealt with which forces her to compensate for it. The compensation was to go into a cocoon.

Tell me more about losing connection, please.

Here is the cocoon again. It is really throughout. It is not a cliché in this case.

"It is a matter of integrity and existing in a full life with laughter, joy and sadness. When I put the coat over my head, it was the last time I could be. It was a way of keeping grounded. I just was."

Pierre: Do you have a fear of downward motion?

And again we have the cocoon.

"How do you know? Yes I do.

Pierre: Because I think I know the remedy you need and the remedy you need is well known in homeopathy to have that fear of downward motion. It is a way of confirming the remedy.

The way she explained the cocoon was, of course, perfect. I say "of course" because as I mentioned before people always say things right. That leads me to a particular point. It is very common for people

REMEDY:

Boron

FOLLOW UP: (One month)

Pierre: How have you been?

"The anxieties have been radically altered, I have much more equilibrium. The anxieties are gone but I am not very focused. It is still difficult to process everything but I am getting there."

Give me a sense of the process since you took the remedy, please.

"The first two weeks after the remedy I felt OK, just being, existing, that felt very good and it still feels that way. I would like to feel like I have a handle on things rather than just being but I feel something changed in my inner core. I am feeling far more relaxed. With harmony and flow it is all much better. Even our daughter seems to be better now. I feel more connected to myself. I am discovering who I am again, I am seeing things more clearly and I am feeling more personally powerful. The gum infection is also better and so is the bursitis in the right shoulder. The shin pain is totally gone. All the pains I had are much better but I still don't feel very grounded in my body. It is better but not completely better."

Clearly this is good, can you tell me more?
"I think I have become less impulsive. The anger I had has changed too, now I am like "whatever..." whereas it used to be a simmering pot. The feeling of being in a

to be concerned about what they say. There is no right or wrong during a homeopathic consultation. The questions are meant to express feeling spontaneously and creatively. The feelings lead to experience.

This remedy relates to the stage of developing *in utero* at the stage in getting engaged. It is one of the stages of being in the "cocoon." She describes it so perfectly well. The fear of downward motion stems from the feeling of not wanting to "come down" from the comfort of the cocoon.

After the remedy she felt she was "existing." She has come out of the cocoon. Existing, is being on her own. She says she would like to have "a handle on things." She still wants to hold on but clearly the feeling is nowhere near as strong as it used to be.

"Even our daughter seems better now." The feeling that other people in our surrounding are better after taking a remedy for one self is common. As our inner Being is tuned up to a healthier state from the lifting of the disorder so does our perception of the world and, reciprocally,

cocoon is much better. All the powerlessness is gone."

REMEDY:

Continue

MORE FOLLOW UPS: (One and a half year)

"I feel well. My anxieties have not been much of a problem at all.

the perception of the world toward us. This is similar to Hillary's case (see Hillary case) of post partum depression and the improvement in her relationship with her mother-in-law.

Throughout this case there wasn't much to say. I think her proximity to her art helped her speak about her inner feelings very easily and freely. It was great.
She continues to be well with repetition of the remedy from time to time.

NATASHA

(Early 40's)

DISCUSSION

MM: LOW LIBIDO

- Anger towards husband
- Spider veins, blood spots
- Splitting nails

Pierre: Please tell me what brings you here.

Ever since I had surgery on my elbow to remove some varix. I have had some swelling in the arm. I had a bunch of blood vessels together that formed this varix on my arm, which I had removed. Now I have a lot of itching and tingling along the scar. Then I developed this great sense of fear that has come over me."

Natasha had surgery on the arm for varix (bunched up blood vessels) on the elbow, some swelling remain. She also has some swelling in the middle finger. She complains of craving fats and sugars and has gained six pounds in the last year.

Tell me about that please?

"I have a difficult marriage. The day after I got married I felt a switch go off. The day after I felt devoid of feelings. I felt asexual, I felt like I wasn't connected. I was not attracted to him and I was not responsive. I felt it was not OK to participate in a sexual act within the confines of my marriage."

Tell me about that please? These open-ended questions give the freedom to answer in whichever way people figure is best. I rarely ask a leading question. There is only one in this book in Mollie's case.

Please continue.

"I am fearful of my temper and of my anger towards my father. He did a lot of things he never should have done. I do not want to have the responsibility of having to take care of children; I could not support them emotionally. A while ago I wanted to stab my husband, I was frustrated like a cat in a corner and showing its teeth. I wanted to lash out at people. I was really hysterical. I could not recognize the real issue in front of me and I had remorse for days."

I appreciate the information you are giving me. Please, tell me more.

"I have several issues:
Issue 1: I try to please everybody.
Issue 2: I am fearful of money, I feel it should not be spent. I feel as if I have to explain myself about money issues to my husband."

Long pause for several minutes.

"I don't like people to cling on me, I find it revolting. It feels like my mother wanted to hurt me. She would smile in front of you and stab you in the back. My father could not give love, and he made sure we would not succeed. He was a vicious person and I have a sense that he was doing it on purpose. Some animals eat their young. I see my father with a knife just cutting us down. It was the Antarctic in our house. My anger can be against anybody."

Please, tell me about your dreams.

"There is a cat eating a dead cat with worms coming out it. Then I see my husband drop out of the window. I feel that's OK. I forget about him and then a beautiful cat flies out of the window."

A pause can last several minutes without anyone saying a word. This silence is most of the time a good thing. One can almost see the brain working things out to get deeper. It can be a time of great depth between the two of us. Sometimes something comes out and sometimes all I get is, "I don't know."

Reading this case one could think of Sylvia's case of mastitis (see case). There are, indeed, some similarities but it is completely different. One big difference is that Sylvia

Do you have any strong food cravings or aversion?

"I have a big thing for chocolate. I also like to have a drink or two."

REMEDY:

Theobroma

FOLLOW UP:

Pierre: How have you been?

"I feel like a flower blooming, whatever you gave me, definitely took the edge off. I am not yelling as much. I have to say, I am at a much more intimate level; much calmer, I am shocked at how much more demonstrative I am. My spider veins seem to be much better, they are not as pronounced, especially on the thighs."

SEVERAL MONTHS LATER:

"I am feeling much calmer. I am not getting angry and I communicate with my husband much better. I cleared out the crap I had accumulated in my apartment for the last 17 years. I find that for the first time in my life I am not angry. The anger towards my father has dissipated. Chocolate craving has lessened. Before my period, my mood is not so dramatic. My arm is much better with the tingling less than 10 percent than it was. The swelling on the middle finger is almost gone. I remember now I could not even make a fist when I first came to see you."

needs her close ones, whereas Natasha does not.

When I gave this remedy, I gave it on old-style information I talk about from time to time such as "aversion to husband," etc. (See Chapter 3 or Keshia's case on migraine). Then in 1996, I was introduced to information from colleagues in India. In 2002 they explained qualities of remedies further. In this remedy there is a sense of attachment and detachment. It is a feeling of being estranged or a deep desire for company born out of attachment or detachment. The "Bombay group" in India have helped homeopathy make enormous progress. Thanks to them, my results are far more systematic. When I speak of the difference between the old and the new methods of case taking, I am talking about the breakthroughs that were instituted by their forward-leaning thinking.

The remedy was repeated four times during a period of six months. She was perfectly well and did not need anything further.

JOHN
(5 yr old)

MC: PDD-NOS

Pierre: Tell me about your son, please.

"I have a long list of things that are not appropriate but my biggest concern with him has to do with social peace. He likes to hit his brother, he is very jealous of him. There are a lot of things he does that are not appropriate for him to do. Also his use of speech and language is totally off subject. Lately, he's been talking about balloons constantly. Everything has to do with balloons, He talks about them absolutely nonstop. Another thing, he likes to hide things all the time. He remembers entire sentences from books. Other minor things are: He doesn't like his hair washed. He likes to lie down on cold tiles."

OK, what else, please?

"At 2 months old he had torticollis on the right side. At 3 months old he had a major cough. At 10 months he had a strep infection, now his tonsils are always enlarged and he has a deep and wet cough."

You mentioned social peace.

"He was the happiest kid before his brother was born. He simply does not want to share anything with his brother. He says he wants to go home all the time. He tells his friends

DISCUSSION

I have specialized in autism for many years. It was by far the most challenging time of my professional career. I tried to probe the depth of it so much that I had a radio show on Autismone.org called "Going within." I learned an enormous amount from these children. The number one lesson I learned is to take all children's cases through the mother's state during pregnancy much as in George's case (see case). Once I understood that, the challenge of these cases became like all others.

My next book is already started and is mainly about autism. There is besides that an array of breakthroughs that compel me to write another book. There is a lot of hope to systematically reverse autism.

The foreword by Marie Hernandez is testimony of what can be done for these children.

It should be said that taking the case through the mother's state during the pregnancy is unconventional but it is by far the most productive. In 80% of the cases the mother can relate this most authentic state. Many people tell me at first that the pregnancy was "normal." "I was happy to be pregnant." Once I ask a little, it is very rare it is absolutely

to go home. When people come to our house he blinks his eyes, tenses his shoulders up and throws his head backward when he is mad. He seems to connect to objects. He likes objects that are very smooth, he feels them and rubs them all the time. It is a comfort to him, it seems to be an attachment with the environment, which makes him feel safe. If he didn't have them I think he would feel lost and alone. It is frightening to him to not have these objects with him. There are other things that are not pleasant with him. He takes me by the throat when he needs something, that's simply not appropriate. He has low muscle tone and he likes routines."

REMEDY:

Hyoscyamus niger

FOLLOW UP:

Pierre: How is John?

"There definitely have been some improvements with his language as well as in social situations. He still wants to leave Michael behind but he also wants to give him more. He wants to give him hugs but he also wants to hurt him. He does seem to be more patient overall and he is not as restless as he used to be. He also used to be and he seems to be more independent. He has had fewer tantrums, which makes being around him much more pleasant. He seems less nervous, he doesn't blink his eyes as much as

so but even then I ask "tell me about happy". The state of pregnancy is not the cause of the autism but it is logical that it is the shortest route to find the primary remedy for the child.

This case stands as an "old case" I arrived at the correct remedy in what I would now consider a haphazard way. It is possible to reverse this condition now on a more consistent and homeopathically relevant way.

Up to now we have some pretty common issues of children with PDD-NOS, I decided to go straight into what the mother mentioned first about "social peace" and acknowledge her instinct.

His jealousy toward his brother may seem common. A little bit of jealousy for a couple of days is okay, but in this case it is continuing at a very high level for a very long time therefore it is significant.

Of course, it is common for children with PDD-NOS to not mix with others but for him it was an unsocial behavior rather than just being in his own world. I thought it was homeopathically significant.

There are some good results so I stayed with the same remedy even though the jealousy

before and he does it less when people are around him. He also stopped grabbing me by the throat. When his cousins come over he is definitely part of the crew now."

did not seem that much better.

REMEDY:

Continue

FOLLOW UP:

Pierre: How has John been?

"That remedy did not help as much this time. It took an edge off but it did not go any further. He has been screaming and crying a lot. His aggressiveness did not improve any further with his brother at all; he can turn on a dime and just wants people to leave. We really have a very hard time with him, we have to watch him all the time because we never know what he is going to do with his brother. He screamed once so loud I thought I had fallen in a wasp nest."

The next follow up reveals that the jealousy is not being addressed. Such a major issue in this case led to change the remedy to HYOSCYAMUS.

REMEDY:

Apis mellifica

FOLLOW UP:

Pierre: I suspect what you are going to tell me is going to be good.

"I like what I see. It's made him much more relaxed. He hits his brother a lot less and his obsessive qualities are also much better. His aggressiveness towards the people he knows

This kind of result seemed perfectly good to me. Continuing on the same track was the best thing to do.

is the same but it is not as often,. He still tells his nanny to go home and he doesn't interact greatly with children. He does not approach them but he does want to be with his cousins. Grinding his teeth at night is also better."

Pierre: What else?

"His schoolwork has dramatically improved. (The mother brought me the daily reports from the teacher.

"Another more interactive day."

"Fun time playing our spatial game."

"So happy he is finally opening up to his friends."

"More and more self-initiating. We're all very excited.")

The schoolwork is so much better than before. Combined with the diminished jealousy that was central from day one this is perfect.

Here is a sample of a teacher's note. "I know I've written to you before but John is doing great. He's been very spontaneous and more focused. What progress! I know other teachers have noticed the same".

REMEDY:

Continue

The remedy was repeated several times and then we lost touch until the mother invited me to an autism meeting she organized.

FOLLOW UP 4 YEARS LATER

"He had two strep throat infections within two weeks. Since then he has been losing focus, he needs to be told repeatedly to do things. He gets upset for littlest things and he seems to be worried."

She reported that he was doing great. One year after that she came back. The anti-social behavior changed totally over time.

We repeated the remedy a few times because the appropriate potency had changed. He is doing well now.

REMEDY:

Repeat the last remedy

JOLLIE

(Early sixties)

DISCUSSION

MC: BREAST CANCER

- Prior history of basal cell carcinoma on nose
- Benign tumor on palate
- Arrhythmia
- GERD

Pierre: Tell me please what brings you here?

At this moment I have a lot of problems. I have reflux that is burning me up in the middle of my throat. It is much worse in the middle of the night. I wake up during the night with burning pains between 2 and 4 a.m. then I go back to sleep and once I wake up in the morning I have burning pain in the throat. Then, if I don't take my medication I have burning all day. I am very irritable, short fuse and angry at myself and at the world. I bite the inside of my mouth all the time, I feel like I want to explode and tell people off. I make enemies because I express my dissatisfaction but when I do that I feel better. I have a lot of reasons to be angry, I've been sick and I have not been treated well. I did what I could but I feel helpless; I can't do anything, why do I have cancer? Why me? I have no control or choice of action. I have had such callous physicians."

I present this case because it reflects the wholistic nature of homeopathy not only in P.E.M. but also in its ability to work with traditional medicine. As I detail in chapter one "Homeopathy explained" the two don't have anything to do with each other but both can work toward a similar goal. To put it simply, it is like plumbing. It really does not have anything to do with carpentry but you need both to make the house. This is the way Jollie looked at it.

It is very common for people to ask these types of questions "Why me?" I so often hear it and I wish I could give an answer that could make everyone feel good but I am afraid I don't have the answer to that nor do I think people really expect an answer.

Tell me about your anger, please.

"I have rage towards politicians, the state of the world, sexual scandals, etcetera. I take all of these things seriously. I have no patience for people who are not qualified to make decisions for us. We are at the mercy of people who can't do the job. They usually say, "We don't do that." Well, why not? When I have a job I do it. I would prefer to not have anything to do with anybody. I really find it revolting. Each job I've had they have asked me to do things dishonestly. I can't sign up on that. Everybody screws up and they get away with it. People like me don't have jobs and these people get away with it. One doctor gave me a medication that killed 48 people. People with power sweep that under the carpet at the expense of people. There will always be people who do bad things, but what is scandalous are the supervisors not correcting the problem. It's a failure of morality and rage comes when I can't do anything. I have great difficulty in believing that humanity can't progress, we know how to stop what is not going to work and yet we still do it. There is no progress or it comes slowly. With my cancer I want to be part of the decision."

She is a groundbreaking professional who was one of the first women to earn an MBA.

Her anger is very noble but as always it is not needed. In this case the anger is an integral part of the cancer. The two can't be dissociated. She comes in for basal cell carcinoma and she talks about sex scandals in politics and dishonest executives. What she describes is really fighting an idealistic fight that cannot be won. Her anger is not only with one doctor, it is everybody. Her situation made me think of Don Quichotte.

REMEDY:

Caesium metallicum

After the remedy she made the best decision regarding medical treatment for her cancer: An accelerated radiation

FOLLOW UP:

Pierre: How are you?

"My palpitations and anxieties have not been as bad. I'm sleeping well. I have not had any GERD whatsoever, no burning in the throat! There are many different problems around me but I am holding up well. I can take things better when they don't go the way I want, I must say what you gave me has helped me handle things very well."

REMEDY:

Continue

SEVERAL FOLLOWUPS LATER:

"I continue to improve and I am getting conventional medicine for the cancer that is going very well."

REMEDY:

Same repeated frequently

2 YEARS LATER:

Pierre: What brings you back?

"I have been well up but now I have a little crisis. I've had a rash on my back for the last three months. It is extremely itchy and it is crusting. It never goes away, I have these thick layers of scabs. It feels much worse if I get it wet so I have to be very careful when I take a shower.

protocol considered experimental in this country at the time. It turned out great. The remedy helped her boost her constitution but also helped her get through serious medical treatment with as minimal side effects as one could have. I am not dogmatic. I don't say you must use only homeopathy. Do what you feel is best for you. I think this is the better way to go because in the end if your conscience is clear whatever happens you won't have any regrets.

If you wonder why she waited three months to come, you are in good company, I too wonder each and every time people do that.

Pierre: How did it start?

"I had an abscess on the shoulder blade and then another. I got an injection in each one of them but it didn't help. It started with what looked like an insect bite. Since I often have skin problems on my back I didn't pay too much attention to it at first but it became progressively more itchy. It has been driving me nuts. I went to see several doctors in the last three month and nobody has been able to do anything about it. It is so extremely uncomfortable, the itching really drives me up the wall."

This is a wonderful situation which confirms to me that the remedy helped get rid of the cancer. We'll never know but if we look at the next follow-up and understand that the central remedy can lift any disorder that arises then the proof is there. Read on.

REMEDY:

Ceasium metallicum

I had several remedies in mind, but I decided to go with the remedy that helped her so remarkably 2 years ago. My reasoning was that the intensity of the skin condition was similar to the intensity of her emotional state with the cancer.

FOLLOWUP: (1 month later)

"The itching is at least 90% better. The lesions are much less severe. I have fewer crusts. Almost more importantly nights have been ok I am not as itchy and I have been catching up on sleep."

She repeated the remedy several times and she has been well since.

REMEDY:

Repeat the remedy

MAT

(Late 70's)

MC: SKIPPING HEART BEATS

- Fluttering
- Pain in the heart
- Palpitations
- Difficulty doing daily tasks
- Edema in the legs

Pierre: Please, tell me what brings you here.

"I have had two open heart surgeries with four bypasses in total. The first one was 28 yrs ago and the other one 10 yrs ago. A few months ago my heart started to flutter and skip beats so much that I had to go to the hospital. Ever since my first surgery 28 years ago I take my pulse several times a day, at times I don't feel it for 2 or 3 seconds but in the hospital it was as long as 4 seconds and that is really scary to me. I also have high blood pressure but I take medication to keep it down. One doctor told me to eat rice every day to keep the blood pressure down, I did it but it is still up."

What else can you tell me?

"I feel some pain in my heart and I have some discomfort in the upper left chest. I also experience some burning but that was worse when I was in the hospital. I can't do what I want to do. I feel quite helpless and depressed about being incapable because of my heart

DISCUSSION

I present this case to show how homeopathy can enhance a conventional medical treatment much as in Mollie's case. This is a case with long standing serious cardiac problems. By the time he came to see me he had exhausted all conventional avenues. The beauty here is that even in such an advanced pathological case homeopathy can be tremendously helpful and his cardiologist who had encouraged him then to come see me was pleased and able to judiciously reduce his medications.

With all the problems this man has, a doctor told him to eat rice? Sometimes I hear things that are really surprising to me.

In the hospital he was given Amiodarone (I.V.) for the fluttering. He says, " It gave me the most trouble." He also was given Coreg, which according to him gave him the feeling that he was having a

problems. At this point, I can get pain in the chest at any moment."

This is a very serious situation, are you in close touch with a cardiologist?

"I am but really there is nothing much they can do. The medication they gave me is killing me a little bit at a time. I am used to medications, I mean when you consider my history it is clear that they have done a lot for me but this is the worst I have been in my whole life. The medication they gave me in the hospital was really bad; I have never felt that bad before. I used to work in the garden and play around with mechanical things. Now I can't do anything. I have fallen into a category and I might as well stay there. My wife works and I feel bad about that. I have to do most of the shopping for the house but even that I can't do so much anymore because of my heart and I have to rely on her. I can't even go to the store and carry the bags lest I get palpitations."

Tell me about "falling into a category". What does it mean? How does it feel?

"Being in a category is a limitation in positive and negative ways. I have the feeling of being controlled. I can only go so far in either direction and at times I laugh at my predicament. I am a deeply religious person and I offer my limitation up to God. I feel I have a purpose with my pains, I offer It up to Jesus or Mary. It's a contribution and an

heart attack. Of course that was rather unsettling to him.

Other medications he currently is taking (some were also given in the hospital) are Lisinopral, Novasc, Corgard and Diovan. In other words, the full panoply of medications.

For those who think that I would not recommend seeing a doctor, hold that thought! Conventional doctors are very helpful for all matters of testing and diagnosis. In fact, they are the only ones who can do it.

One big problem I see is that people don't want to tell their doctor when they are taking a homeopathic remedy. I always encourage dialogue even if they are expecting and often get a dose of skepticism.

He offers his pains and his limitations up to Jesus or Mary. What he is explaining is that suffering is a gift to him that he accepts and in turn gives it back as a testament of faith to Mary or Jesus.

exhilaration. When we gain these graces then it comes back three times more. It's my God bank. I am happy to achieve that goal. It is a feeling of success that it will enhance me for eternity."

Could you please tell more about that?

"There is happiness in achieving something. It is like reaching a goal but I accept the limitation and I work within it. Doing well is achieving the best situation. The more good things are done the more are put in a good place and the more it is going to enhance you for eternity. My situation reminds me of the woman in "Moonstruck." It is a situation where a decision needs to be made to achieve the best possible result within the given limitation. It is a challenge."

He is not talking about achieving "the best" but rather the best possible. That is either a dose of reality or a dose of limitation. It is a distinction that makes a difference. Accuracy is tantamount in homeopathy because I need to understand the physical pain in the gestalt of the whole situation.

Could you tell me more about achieving the best possible, please?

"Good is achieving the best situation possible and then having to accept it. There is nothing that I can't control. It's like if a job is lost another can be found. There is no depression this way because you are always betting on the right horse."

Tell me about the experience of being in a situation like in "Moonstruck", please.

"It is a situation of trying to get her happiness back and then accept it. The brother has no right to happiness because he lost his hand. It

Trying and then accepting is a coping mechanism. For the purpose of finding a homeopathic remedy it is absolutely crucial to understand how the person is dealing with the disorder. There are many different kinds; this book brings quite a few to the fore.

is a challenging situation and decisions have to be made to get the best results.

REMEDY:

Tantalum metallicum

FOLLOW UP: (one month later)

Pierre: How are you feeling?

"I am feeling so much better. The doctor took me off two medications, Novasc and Amiorodarone but I am still taking three medications. After the remedy it seemed as if the heart was more stable and able to handle daily stress. It really has made me feel better. I am so much more capable of doing things on my own. The medication was making me feel numb. I am not back to where I was but I feel about 80% better."

As soon as the doctor heard that he was feeling better he took him off Amiorodarone, which was taken in pill form once he was out of the hospital.

I love this case for one simple reason. This man's cardiac history is long and serious. Although no one would say that he could recover totally, the astonishing results this case provides are a great testament as to how the medical and the alternative worlds can work harmoniously together.

REMEDY:

Continue. Repeated the remedy at different intervals over a few months.

SEVERAL FOLLOW UPS: (Several months later)

Pierre: "How are you feeling?"

"Yesterday, the heart started jumping all over the place. There is a feeling of tightness. It is quite scary. At times it feels as if death is imminent. I know the feeling well. I've had it in the past. I repeated the remedy, I feel better but not a great deal like before."

At times, he feels like death is imminent. As I mentioned before, his cardiologist follows him very closely. He figured he would not wait and he asked me if there was anything he could take to relieve the tightness and the erratic heartbeat.

REMEDY:

Aconitum napellus 12C or 30C

FOLLOW UP: (two weeks later)

Pierre: "How are you?"

"The Aconitum you gave me helped in the *30C* potency, the *12C* didn't help at all. I feel I went through quite a moment since I was feeling like I could have a heart attack at any time. I still feel like I am recovering from all the medications they gave me in the hospital months ago. I feel I am more stable than I have been in a long time."

I recommended the remedy Aconitum (when feeling scared of an imminent heart attack, it is one of the few indicated) and to continue with the constitutional remedy.

I don't list the potency I give in the book because it is not needed to understand homeopathy. In this case it is important to make the distinction because the situation is really acute.

Aconitum was repeated several times.

PHONE CALL:

Pierre: How are you feeling?

"I am feeling well, I am continuing with the remedy. I don't have any need for anything but I would like to get my blood pressure under control without medications. Even the edema I had ever since the second surgery got better. My level of activity is better. I can carry packages and I can even dance a little. I feel about 90%."

I recommended that going too far without medication was not my goal. I didn't want to push the envelope.

Two months later he reported he was holding off the remedy because he was feeling well. I don't know if he ever got off the other medications. To me that was not the goal. My goal was a good life free of cardiac symptoms and anxieties about his heart issues. That much was achieved.

REMEDY:

Continue

ARTHUR

(4 yr old)

DISCUSSION

MC: COUGH

• Asthma

Pierre: What is happening with your child?

Mother: "He has this horrible cough and his eyes are always tearing. Can you tell me why his eyes get better in the cold?

I don't know. I could give you a lot of "reasons" that would sound good but really no one knows, Please tell me about the cough.

"Between the ages of 1 and 2 he didn't get anything, he did not get sick or anything. Then he started to have eczema around his mouth. The skin became dry and lighter in the area. After that, a couple of weeks ago he got croup. He was wheezing and gasping for air. It was very difficult to see him like this. The doctor gave him a steroid medication and he kind of got better. Then he got sick again and he got steroids again but we don't think he should be on steroids."

Is this what is going on now?

"No, now he has had a cold ever since he had the croup. He doesn't have any fever, his nose is running and the mucus is yellowish green."

"Can you tell me why his eyes get better in the cold?" the mother asked. These questions can't be answered truthfully. To me this is just a symptom that should fit in within the whole picture. It is what is called throughout this book an SRP. Strange, Rare and Peculiar). Indeed, many "reasons" could be given that would sound logical and make people feel good but no one really knows. Finding the remedy is the only truth to me.

Could you describe the cough, please?

"He coughs every morning around 5 AM. It is a wheezing cough. Whenever he runs around he has short bursts of DRY cough. The doctors only want to give him steroids but there must be something better. He is not himself. He complains that he is very hot, he wants to open the windows all the time. He is annoyed, irritated and short tempered. At the same time, he looks for sympathy. He wants to be held all the time. He doesn't want to be put down. He doesn't want to eat anything or drink anything. He just wants to sip some water."

REMEDY:

Pulsatilla. Call me tomorrow

PHONE: (next day)

"He is not better"

REMEDY:

Spongia tosta

It is not in the nature of this child to want to be held so wanting to be held and looking for sympathy become qualities that should be considered as the way he is being affected. Yet, most children want to be held when they are not feeling well. It's a bit of a quandary but since there were no other qualifying attributes I decided on the remedy Pulsatilla.

ONE DAY LATER:

Pierre: How is it going?

Mother: "He slept the whole night. He didn't cough and woke up at 12PM. The short bursts of cough are gone. Usually when he is sick he is restless but this time he slept very well. His watery eyes are totally better."

The remedy Spongia tosta acted very well and his condition improved a lot overnight. The parents repeated the remedy a few times

FOLLOW UP: (4 months later)

Pierre: It has been a little while.

Mother: "He has been well ever since we last saw you but he coughed all night. His eyes have been watery for a couple days. He is scratching them too; they seem to be itchy. Now he has a barking cough. The cough is not as dry as it used to be. He does not like the heat. I gave Spongia but it didn't do anything this time."

That was a good decision. Try to tell me more about him now.

"I noticed he seems to get sick after he has a problem in school. He was very agitated last week. He was breathing differently. I never noticed this before but then again I never paid attention to these things before I started with homeopathy."

Pierre: What other observations have you made?

"I don't know, His watery and itchy eyes seem to be the most important symptom I see right now. They have been like that for a couple of days."

REMEDY:

Euphrasia

during the week. They were watching for symptoms such as either getting hot with or without fever or watery eyes. If either happened the remedy was repeated. Wait and observe is the best way to go about repeating a remedy. In a situation like this, there is no need to automatically repeat the remedy. What is important is to watch the signs of the Vital Force and act accordingly. There is great order in the disorder one could say. Symptoms don't occur out of the blue but rather in order.

Here we have the eye symptoms again.

"I never paid attention to the details of symptoms before." This is a very interesting comment. People do observe more acutely once they start homeopathy. I believe that that alone is a substantial benefit towards knowing one's body more deeply.

I have to admit that I overlooked the remedy Euphrasia for a cough. His watery eyes led me to feel a tug on my shirt and look it up in the *Materia Medica*. I was pleasantly surprised to see that most of the symptoms listed for it in the MM fit the cough very well. Euphrasia is well known for its eye symptoms, particularly for allergies. In

PHONE:

"The cough and the watery eyes have completely cleared up."

fact, the common name of Euphrasia is eye bright.

It never ceases to amaze me as to how deep the MM really is. Every time I read about a remedy, I discover something "new" about it. It is a daily and endless quest for perfection.

JUANITA
(4 yrs old)

DISCUSSION

MC: RECURRING COUGH

- Reactive airway disorder
  - Frequent colds

I present this case because sometimes unbeknown to them people can even tell me what the remedy needed is. In this case the mother made a very astute observation for her child.

Pierre: Please tell me what is going on?

Mother: "She catches colds very easily and she has great difficulty breathing. She is getting oral steroids. She started sneezing in March (2 months ago) then in April her nose started to run. Her cold doesn't seem to go away. She has been getting one ear infection after another. She got better after we used the nebulizer but three weeks later the sneezing and coughing started again. Her congestion seems to be worse at night. She starts to breathe faster and faster. The breathing became so fast we had to go to the emergency room."

Could you please give me some of her history?

When courses of antibiotics are given over and over again the inner balance causing the problem is not addressed and the disorder keeps on recurring because it is fundamentally not removed.

"She has had 4 ear infections in the last 5 months treated with four courses of antibiotics. We can't keep going this way. We can't keep giving her antibiotics and wait for the next time it happens and do the same thing again."

Please tell me how it develops.

"Usually she gets a runny for a few days and then she develops a fever. Once she gets a fever she becomes very quiet. She asks for milk or water and stays quiet. Her face gets flushed and she sweats on the head. At the same time she gets a little constipated and the stool gets very dry. After the fever starts she begins to breathe through her nose very quickly."

Can you tell me what the breathing sounds like?

The breathing sounds "tinny" as in tin coming from her system. I can't explain it; her abdomen goes in and out very quickly. She was diagnosed with Reactive Airway Disorder. We feel we must do something else."

REMEDY:

Stannum

FOLLOW UP:

"She didn't cough all night. We repeated the remedy the next day and she got completely better. One week later she got a cold. She coughed a bit during the night and then better during the day. Now she is well, she doesn't cough and she does not have breathing problems."

AUTHOR'S COMMENT:

Another recommendation I make is to limit milk intake during the winter. If you have a child who gets colds, coughs and ear

I always ask parents what the breathing sounds like. This was the first time I ever got an answer that was point on. Most of the time people say it is a deep cough. It is very unusual to have parents totally nail an observation like that. From the homeopathic point of view it is the essence. We have lost our sense of observation; it would be good to gain it back. Stannum is actually the homeopathic remedy of tin. From the observation of the mother we arrived at the remedy.

Speaking as a father, I offer two recommendations as follows: Children don't like to be covered at night yet when I ask what the child or baby wears the answer is usually "a pajama." That is not enough. I recommend putting on several overalls at night. We layer during the day, why not at night? As adults, we sleep snuggly under several blankets yet the child has one pajama so of course they're getting sick, they're not covered enough.

infections, give up the milk during the winter months and see your child thrive. This is outside the homeopathic realm but from one parent to another it will do wonders for your child's ears. You can replace milk with any of the alternatives available, most of them rich in calcium.

SERGIO
(7 yr old)

DISCUSSION

MC: ANGER
• Allergies
• Night sweats

Pierre: What brings you here with this child?

Mother: "He is aggressive. He smacks kids. He spits. He goes blind when he is upset and he can't stop. He just goes after a kid."

Wow, who would have thought?

"Yes, he is also very cynical. He makes noises all day long. 'Oh, hah, yah yah yah.' He hums all day long too. He will provoke a child when he doesn't know him."

Please, tell me more.

"He confronts us all the time, too. Physically, he sweats so much at night when he falls asleep that we sometimes have to change his pajamas during the night. He has allergies, his nose is stuffed and he sleeps with his mouth open."

Please continue. Tell me more about him.

"He ignores everybody. He doesn't respect the teacher or anybody. He just continues to do his thing. It is always a struggle to do something. He does not share his toys and yet he takes toys from other children. He gets

This case is amazing in the amount of time a total turn around happened. Within a matter of days this child returned to being a well-behaved kid. Best of all it happened 100% naturally. While homeopathy can be extraordinarily fast, expecting such rapidity is not realistic.

This child's behavior is truly out-of-bounds. Although in this case there is not much to defend, most parents give a lot of excuses for their children's deeds and actions. As much as it is an unenviable

into this rage, goes blind and just wants to hit. Last week he totally unloaded on a child. He doesn't stop until he's taken away no matter how big the other child is. Even when there is a new kid, he starts to provoke that kid, he pushes and kicks and then, of course, he is left on the side by himself. That is exactly what happened at the pool the other day."

What else can you tell me about him besides his behavior? Is there anything unusual that he mentions frequently or complains about frequently?

"He is very sensitive to noises, he just doesn't like noise. He also has a very restless sleep. There is one other thing; since he was 4 or 5 years old he feels his heart beat, he talks to me about it all the time."

REMEDY:

Theridion

FOLLOW UP: (1month)

Mother: "He's been very good. The rage has totally disappeared. He is so much better. We don't have to battle over everything, he is a lot more responsive. He was making noises before but now it is also totally gone. He is doing his homework well. At this moment we could not be any happier. Even the sweat when he falls asleep is almost gone."

Pierre: I would really like to encourage you to keep up with the follow-ups please because

situation for them and the child, at this point we have only general behaviors about his raging conduct rather than individualizing characteristics; there is nothing, so far, upon which I can suggest a remedy accurately.

At this point, I had asked questions for close to two hours. I had an idea of the category of remedies I should be looking into but I was quite at a loss as to what I could specifically recommend.

The two slivers of information that "he is very sensitive to noise" and "he hears his heart beat all the time" gave me enough keynotes upon which I could confidently propose a remedy. This is the old-fashioned form of analysis whereby picking what we call strange, rare and peculiar (SRP) reveals the remedy rather than having a narrative that weaves perfectly from beginning to end to give a perfect understanding of the remedy needed. I had to fall back on a more mechanical way of figuring the remedy out.

we need to make sure we build on this base rather than wait for a setback.

NOTE:

Several months later he had a slight relapse. Considering the way he potentially is if he were to fully relapse, the parents brought him back. The remedy was repeated in the same potency and the remedy had no effects. It surprised me to no end and I practically retook the case right then and there. I could not find where I had gone wrong so I repeated the remedy again in a different potency and right away he improved and has been well since. To this day it remains a mystery as to why that happened.

I have also seen both parents and neither has been very diligent at keeping up regular visits which is very necessary, particularly in the first six months to a year. The better we do at the beginning the better the results for the long term are possible.

DANIEL

(6 months old)

MC: ECZEMA

• Allergies

Pierre: What is going on with this baby?

Mother: "He has eczema on his arms with lesions on his legs, his face and his back. The eczema is definitely aggravated by bathing and we noticed that milk clearly affects him for the worse."

When did this start?

"He's always had very bad reflux. We started him on formula after 1 month because I did not have breast milk. He never slept well at night, waking and crying and vomiting all the time. He always wanted continuous nursing; the first week was difficult he was not latching on properly so I was pumping instead. I had a lot of difficulties building a supply up, then he went on a nursing strike and after that I had to have surgery for a herniated disk. As if this were not enough, he went on strike again. Now he has been taking the bottle OK."

Wow, I admire the effort you put into trying to breastfeed. Tell me more about him.

"He started sleeping badly after my mother-in-law stopped helping. She had to go back home. Since then he has not been the same. We started dealing with his allergies about a

DISCUSSION

This case shows the importance of the state of the mother during pregnancy. I am proud to say I've had breakthroughs in this matter that should help any child improve substantially. The issues in this case may seem mundane but they are real and central to his eczema.

Here is a non-homeopathic recommendation to mothers who "don't have enough milk" and want to lower the chances of mastitis or, better yet, want to avoid colic in their babies.
Make a tea:
3 cups of water:
1teaspoon grounded fennel seeds.
1teaspoon grounded fenugreek.
1teaspoon Anise seeds.
Optional.
1teaspoon Grounded caraway seeds.
The first 3 items are available in most grocery store. Let steep for ½ hour.
You can find these teas online already made or try Weleda Nursing tea, which is more

month ago. His eyes became very red and he was sneezing but he didn't have a runny nose at the time. Now he is itching because of the eczema on his scalp and ears. We swaddle him in his blanket very tightly so that he doesn't scratch his arms and legs. It is really difficult to see."

Could you tell me about the pregnancy, please?

"Everything went fine during the pregnancy except that I felt very anxiety ridden. I was worried much more than usual. I felt isolated here. We may be moving back home. I am having many difficulties with my husband. I have taken a leave of absence from my job and am planning to quit. Any normal routine here is out of the window"

Please, would tell me about being worried?

"My husband and I get into some pretty big arguments. I was worried about my job, my marriage; I had nausea and a back problem. I could not get things done, which worried me even more. I obsessed and read medical information online about ultra sound, amniocentesis. I would go over it a lot, doing all this reading very anxiously. I felt like I was stuck in a rut, totally overwhelmed. I have been in a rut my whole life. I am going around in circles, I have been feeling so inadequate, and I feel bad, sad and unhappy."

readily available. Ideally, purchase the tea before the baby is born and start drinking it right after birth and each day thereafter. You will always have enough milk and the baby will have a much less chance of having colic. If the mother doesn't have enough milk, then a homeopathic remedy is needed for her but keep in mind that 98% of Swedish women breastfeed, they are no different than American women or Western European women whose statistics say only 50% breast feed.

By understanding the mother's state during the pregnancy we are able to understand the inner state of the disorder of the baby. In Curt's case of food allergies (see case) right after this one, I talk about Vital Heredity (VH).

Could you tell me the opposite feeling of the way you are feeling now?

"The opposite feeling is that of being close to someone, loving. It's a warm feeling; it's a physical sensation that reminds me what it was like when I was a child, close to a few people that somehow was comforting to me. As a child, when the summer came it was the best time. I didn't have pressure on me. I spent time with my brother and sisters going to the beach, feeling comforted and cared for. Going to the beach, I felt connected to my family. I feel no affection at all now and that is the biggest problem I have."

I tried many different ways to find out about the deeper feelings rather than the broad ones she mentions such as "going around in circles" or "feeling inadequate" but I could not get any deeper. So, I asked for the opposite feeling of what she was not able to explain which is really the other side of the same coin.

Please tell me about your dreams.

"I have great dreams. There usually is a party; a family type of party, a wedding type and everybody is having a great time. I always feel great after I dream. It is a very warm feeling."

Is it a similar feeling as you described to me before?

"I really want to go back home. I feel over there everything will come back to normal. It is the same feeling. I never thought about that before."

REMEDY:

Magnesium Muriaticum

The theme of family we see in this case seems banal and logical but when you read the cases in this book you see that in the end she could have related the same feeling to anything else. In other words, any disorder would have spurred a similar experience or perception to the one she has now. The perception is the essence of the disorder here.

FOLLOW UPS: (Generally on the phone.)

Pierre: How has he been?

"He has been much better. The eczema on the arm and the patches on the leg are gone. The itching is much better. His reflux is much better. He had some sneezing and coughing but not that frequent at all. He still wakes up frequently, he nurses (bottle) and goes back to sleep. This is a major difference from before."

How about you, how are you doing?

"The feeling of isolation has diminished greatly and there is definitely an improvement in my relationship with my husband. I am not getting any more done than before, but I am not feeling stuck. I'm feeling very relaxed and comfortable with myself. I'm not going back to work as soon as I thought and I am not as worried as I normally would be."

MORE FOLLOW UPS:

"He has not been fussy. He rarely cries and the reflux is gone. He seems fine in all aspects. A little dryness on the forearms remains, that's all."

Family is a universal feeling. In this case it is central. Even the dreams are about family gatherings. For example, I am from France. My family lives there but I am perfectly happy here in the U.S. I do not suffer from it. In this case, going back would relieve her problems temporarily to a small degree but it would not solve the eczema. Only the proper remedy can do that.

What is truly fascinating in this case is that the baby (6 months old) reacted once the mother-in-law stopped helping. Is it a loss of family? Perhaps. Certainly from the point of view of homeopathy it is transference of the Vital Force (VF). When she mentions "a warm feeling," she is feeling family, not a lover, not her husband (although it would help to not have arguments). She wants family as there is at a wedding (dreams), or at the beach (childhood).

I asked to dilute one pellet in a little bit of water and to give the baby a sip. The instruction was to look out for itching. If the itching subsides do not repeat. If the itching starts again give another sip.

I also told the mother to take one dose of the remedy and she improved successfully as well.

CURT

(8 months old)

DISCUSSION

MC: ECZEMA

• Violent reaction to food

Pierre: Could you please tell me as much as you can about the eczema?

Mother: "He has had this eczema for the last 4 months. He had to be hospitalized for a violent reaction to soy. There was a pool of vomit. He had shallow breathing, we didn't know what to do and we called the ambulance. It was really bad."

It sounds like a difficult and traumatic time, I am very sorry to hear that.

"He's also been sick for 3 weeks and his nose has been congested ever since then. The heat in the apartment makes him worse. His face breaks out and it gets irritated particular on the margin of his hair. That's actually where the whole thing started."

What else can you tell me, please?

"For the last two nights he has been really bad but at first the skin started to break on the cheeks, then on the forehead, especially between the eyebrows and in the crease of the arms, hands and wrists, then behind the knees, down the legs on the shin, calf and ankles. In general, his left side breaks out more than the right and now it's moving up the chest. The skin breaks. He wakes up itching

Eczema, in my view, is not a skin condition but rather an allergic reaction.

I present this case because many children suffer from eczema. A lot of creams are applied but the skin is an organ so if it is suppressed the problem will go deeper. In most of these cases the skin allows discharge serving as an outlet in a way to maintain health in the deeper structures of the body. When the VF (Vital Force) is no longer able to exhibit the symptoms on the superficial level, the next level of weakness is generally respiratory.

I asked many more questions but I could not elicit more physical descriptions than that. This was a very long time ago and today, as you might have seen in other children's cases, I ask about the mother's state during the pregnancy. The fact that

at night around 2 a.m. He sucks on his hands to the point of his skin cracking. I have had something similar to that for years, myself."

REMEDY:

Petroleum

FOLLOW UP: (phone one week later)

"He improved for a short time and now he is the same as before. At this moment, it looks as if nothing has changed.

REMEDY:

Upon remembering the skin of the mother (mainly dry and breaking), I changed the remedy to *Sarsaparilla.*

FOLLOW UP: (1 month later)

"He has been much more tolerant of food such as dairy, wheat, oats, corn and rice. We still stay away from soy but the legs have completely cleared, as well as the ankles and the chest. He still scratches his hands but not as much. The skin is returning to normal now, it had gotten so thick I felt pain just looking at it. When the dog licks him he does not turn red any more. He still has a few little cracks behind the ears and hands, but for the most part his skin has almost completely cleared."

MORE FOLLOW UPS:

"He continues to strive and be better than he ever was."

she has a similar skin condition further validates that approach. This is what I call Vital Heredity (VH) as in Daniel's case of eczema. Certainly heredity exists. It is obvious to everyone. We all experience it and see it in ourselves, friends and family. The great thing here is that we can do something about it. We are not "doomed," as some would like to have us believe, to the whims of our genes.

The remedy was close, it had some resonance because he improved for a short time but it is not accurate enough for longstanding improvement.

After changing the remedy, he has needed repetition of the remedy only a few times for small outbreaks after certain foods.

This very early case shows the great variation between cases then and now. Today's information is thoroughly deep, lively and reflects the human experience. This case shows few of the deeper feelings. The difference is like the difference between watching a black and white versus a color TV.

One last thing: Don't you love the dog licking part of this case?

STEVE	DISCUSSION
(11 yr old)	

MC: WARTS
- Nightmares
- Dryness of skin

Pierre: How can I help you?

Mother: "He has warts! They first started on the knees but he also has some on his thumbs, fingers, knees, on his back and in his armpit for over a year. The doctor burned a couple of them off but they keep coming back. He has dry skin, all these small white excrescences are sensitive to touch. He gets at least one new wart every month."

I can see on the hands there are quite a few. What more can you tell me?

"He has a history of allergies to strawberries. He has had several ear infections and his nose is constantly running. Look at his upper lip; it is irritated all year round, it is always red."

Steve, what can you tell me about your skin? How does it feel?

Steve: "The cold weather makes my skin very dry; it feels as if it makes ice on my skin. I feel piercing ice on my face, so much so that at times I scream from pain."

Mother: "Several years ago, he had pain during urination. He said it was as if a knife was cutting him. He even had some pain

"He has warts!" besides that there are not enough details and there wasn't anything uncommon to them. Like most conditions, the deeper levels need to be understood and therefore properly addressed with the remedy to restore order on the physical level.

Rather than just burning the warts, homeopathy seeks to restore inner balance at the Vital Force level so that the dry skin, the warts and the nightmares disappear, as you will see later. There is no difference between the conscious state and subconscious. There isn't a wall separating the two. The P.E.M. are connected as well and the beauty of homeopathy is that we can navigate all the different levels in order to arrive at the most correct remedy. All of them have one thing in common: they all hold a piece of the root of disorder.

I very often talk about strange, rare and peculiar

when he went swimming in the ocean. He was under the control of this pain, as if a little demon were inside him. The whole body was disturbed, all the limbs were moving in different directions. It was as if someone had pricked him and he became someone else."

Tell me about your dreams, please.

Mother: "He has very frightful dreams."

Steve: "I look at an object and I think it's someone. I am afraid of being alone. Very often I feel nervous and scared. I always feel as if there is a glass ball in my stomach. I also feel as if there is a hollow spot in my body like there is something pushing my intestines around and it doesn't feel right. If I close my eyes and hear some noise, I feel as if someone wants to kill me. I remember a dream; I see a small pink elephant and I can't fall asleep. In the dream, my father screams at me and he takes it away from me to put it in the garbage. I feel as if I am in space. I hear my father, calm but upset. The floor is up on the side and I feel as if I am floating, as if the whole world has something against me for a small thing. I feel as if people are watching me. In my dreams, I often feel like I need to do something, so that the girl is going to like me. I feel as if I would be detested if I do something small."

Does he complain of stomach problems sometimes?

Mother: "Yes, he does, but I never thought anything of it."

(SRP) symptoms. "The cold weather makes me feel like it is piercing the skin to the point of screaming" is exactly that.

Although there seems to be a wealth of SRP information here, unfortunately it turned out to not be very useful. Further questioning didn't bring more details.

In teenage cases, it can be quite challenging to get deeper homeopathically meaningful information. On to the dreams...

This child related his dreams in wonderful details and feelings. He has a lot of fear about his father accompanied by a feeling of weakness towards him. The father could be the most wonderful dad in the world, but in the dream it is his perception. It is his perception on the subconscious level. Keep in mind, this is not psychotherapy. We just use what it homeopathically relevant.

He is not coping well and he is weaker, which, in his case, makes him feel like he is in outer space. He is not fitting in his body, or he is not quite here on the earth plane. This is the essence of the remedy I gave. It is also a well-known remedy for warts.

REMEDY:

Thuja occidentalis

FOLLOW UP: (1 month later)

Pierre: Is he feeling better?

Mother: "He has had far fewer nightmares and it's been a lot easier for him to fall asleep. He is also much calmer and he controls himself better. He has not mentioned anything about his fears of someone wanting to kill him or follow him. After I saw you, I thought about it and I realized he mentioned someone was following him or wanting to kill him just about every day. It is amazing to see the warts literally disappear. There is only one wart on the left finger, which is much smaller. The warts between the fingers are gone. The ones on his legs are still there but new ones don't seem t be coming out anymore."

Pierre: How is the stomach?

Steve: "The ball in my stomach is gone. Also I don't see my body from a bird's eye view. I think it is 90 percent better."

Mother: "I also noticed he has much less anger over little things."

REMEDY:

Wait

This remedy is often given only based on the warts, but once it is given based on PEM then it becomes a certainty that it is the correct remedy.

It is interesting that we see an impression in the stomach as there is in the dream, namely that of being made of glass.

In the dream he was in space, outside his body. Awake he was seeing his body from a bird's eye view. This is really the same feeling. I always find The Golden Thread of the VF (Vital Force) extremely interesting. I never cease to be amazed! More important than being amazed, we can do something about the whole problem at once by matching the dynamic remedy to the dynamis of the person.

FOLLOW UP: (3 months later)

Mother: "The warts are all gone. The ball in the stomach and hollow spot are all gone. The dry skin on the cheeks and the crusty eczema are all gone. He is much calmer than before. He wasn't restless before at all but there was an edge that I no longer see in him. He seems much better in his own skin."

Steve: "My concentration in school is much better; I am not daydreaming like before and I fall asleep quickly."

"He is better in his own skin." Considering the case, one could say that indeed!

SANDRA
(Mid 30's)

DISCUSSION

MC: CHRONIC TONSILLITIS
- Cold sores
- Frequent colds
- Hair loss

Pierre: Tell me about your chronic tonsillitis, please.

"It started as far back as when I was a young child. My husband seems to think it has been worse since I gave birth. I have to admit that it is almost always there. Sometimes it is followed by a nagging dryness in the throat and an itching cough. I have had a lot of hair loss since the pregnancy. Combined with a low immune system, I am getting frequent colds so it has been difficult. Even when my throat is normal, my tonsils look like a mess."

Please, describe how it starts and develops a little more.

"When I get tonsillitis I first feel tired. It is like I am turning a low-grade fever on just like you turn an oven on. I don't get a fever each time but it feels like it, then I feel tension in my throat, and later the scratching begins. It becomes very difficult to swallow and the pain goes to the ear. After that I get a fever within one day."

Right off the bat she takes the whole problem back to childhood. This is significant. Considering the main complaint of tonsillitis, which homeopathically is considered superficial, it may mean that the Vital Force (VF) has not weakened into a deeper disorder.

Her husband makes the interesting and uncommon observation for a husband that "her tonsillitis has been worse since she gave birth." Had the husband been there I would have asked him more about it.

You know the development of the tonsillitis very well, please, tell more.

"Well, after that the throat feels tight and it swells, it becomes difficult to swallow and my tongue becomes coated. At that point it begins to take all my attention. I get concerned about whether I am going to get sick. Is it going to progress into something or not? On the first day of feeling like that, I may have a chance to get better if I get a lot of sleep. Every time I am going to get sick it worries me. "Here we go again." The situation really frustrates me. If I am involved in some activity I may not feel it as badly as it really is but it does not stop it and then I pay the price for not paying attention to it."

Please tell me about it "taking all your attention."

"It just does. A person should do what they are supposed to do. It takes all my attention. Instead of flowing, it is right there. Out of 100 units of attention it takes 90 like I am my throat. Then I wonder, is it going to progress into something worse? What is contributing to this? Can I get more sleep? I get very wrapped up in it. My whole life I have been getting this and it concerns me. Another thing, I have been getting cold sores if I am out in the sun. There is something defective in me. It is as if I bought a brand new car and there is something wrong with it; I got gypped on my tonsils and my mouth."

When someone describes their symptoms well, the best thing to do is to let them speak freely and unobtrusively. The flow is very important. One can have faith that most of what is needed will be told with minimal questioning. It is like in Samuel's case (see case) of PTSD; there was little to ask. It should be pointed out that this is rare. Most of the time the questions are repetitive and difficult or frustrating to answer.

The way she describes her condition is very lively. She has had this condition for so long she really knows it well. She really embodies the condition.

What is the feeling of being gypped?

"I don't want these body parts. I don't want them, they are not supposed to be working this way, and I am lacking the data to do something about it. Sometimes people feel that when something is going on it has to do with somebody else. That's not accurate, I have this imperfect body part and I want to reclaim it. My throat and mouth are not supposed to be this way. It is a mystery to me, I look for answers inwardly but I don't get anywhere. I can recall when I was a child what I wanted to do. As a child I had certainty about the path I wanted to take and two family members were critical of that. It shook up the certainty I had. That's when my tonsils started acting up."

Tell me more about how you felt then, please.

"Someone in my family was criticizing me. I remember it was a destabilizing feeling. I was very aware as a child and there was a lot of unhappiness. I was very communicative. I knew I could produce good results; I wanted to be an artist. I did not have much doubt about my abilities. Before being criticized, I felt very solid and directed. Now I'm shaken up and I'm just holding on to what I know. It's a struggle to hold on to what I know. It's a wobbly path."

This is wonderful information for my purpose. Please continue.

"Of course, it didn't help when my mother-in-law was talking about me either. She was

"Lacking data." The language is wonderfully squarely expressive. Throughout the interview she is making very square gestures, her hands are parallel to each other going up and down. This points to structure, which is similar to Roger's case of numbness (see case) in the hands and can indicate an element/mineral type of remedy. The expression of the VF is reflected at all levels. Everything that is said is all Truth.

As a child she had "certainty" and then someone said something "that shook her up."

She was "very communicative" and then got "shaken up" and since then she has had throat problems. This is not a case for psychotherapy, not a case for antibiotics. It is not psychosomatic either. It is a case for homeopathy. It is interesting to note that she wanted to be an artist. An artist is all about expression and she has throat problems. An artist is often someone who attracts attention and

critical of my pursuits. That really made me feel insecure or shaken up about it again."

Tell me about feeling "shaken up," please.

"It is not knowing. It is very uncomfortable and you just hold on to what you know. You harness it in some way. It is a struggle to hold on to what you know because at the same time you have a few doubts about that. It is a wobbly path."

REMEDY:

Argentum metallicum

FOLLOW UP: (One and two months)

Pierre: Have you have been better?

"The first week was a little difficult. The mucus in the nose increased along with the eye discharge. Then for 3 or 4 days, I had intense intestinal cramping, as if a rock was trying to go through. After that I developed a dry itching cough and now my tonsils are definitely smaller. The right one acts up a little more than the left but it doesn't take my attention as much as before."

Good start. What else can you tell me?

"The feeling of worry has reduced dramatically. I don't worry about my throat getting sore and I feel a lot more stable."

this is exactly what she says about the tonsillitis. Isn't it fascinating? I just love this. I ask totally open-ended questions and the answers lay out the correct remedy right before me. All there is left for me to do is to give it.

Now she is going back to "hold on" which is the same word she used as when she was speaking of reclaiming her body part.

The homeopathic remedy is very clear at this point. Indeed it is an element.

A slight increase in symptoms can occur, although it rarely happens in my practice. In this case throughout the years she had used a lot of antibiotics, perhaps the remedy was helping cleanse that at first. It could also be that the potency was not 100% exactly precise for her.

SEVERAL FOLLOW-UPS LATER: (Over two years)

"I have been doing very well. My son and husband are sick right now but I have not gotten sick. Usually when that happens I get a full-blown throat infection. My tonsils are not so swollen. Actually under normal circumstances the tonsils are OK. I don' have a low-grade fever. My hair has stopped falling out. I'm happy."

Her physical complaints and her emotional level are much better. One could say, "Well, of course she is better emotionally, it is logical since the physicals are better." Well, not so fast. All these years she took antibiotics didn't make her feel better so deeply. Now, because the remedy acts upon the totality, the deeper effects are bearing fruit on all levels for greater health to occur and eventually prevail.

CYNTHIA
(Early 40's)

MC: CROHN'S DISEASE

- Gall bladder stones
- Tubercular peritonitis

Pierre: Please, tell me as much as you can about your Crohn's disease.

"I developed a fistula on the scar of the surgery when I was in college. That was bad. Now, two years ago, the Crohn's started to act up again. I started acupuncture treatment, which did not give me any relief. I went to see a nutritionist, that didn't help and after that I saw a homeopath who gave me *Phosphorus LM1 up to LM6* without any long-lasting effects. He then changed the remedy to *Arsenicum album LM1-2* but I still didn't get any relief. Now, I am taking medication but it only relieves a little bit and the Crohn's must be getting worse because I feel like I am going into a relapse."

OK, please tell me as much about the Crohn's as you can.

"I don't think I tolerate stress very well. I was fine after the peritonitis until I was 33 or 34 years old. I was hospitalized again at 39 because of another abdominal fistula. At 41, I was hospitalized again for the fistula in the same location as before. My liver enzymes

DISCUSSION

Cynthia was diagnosed with Crohn's disease at the early age of 13 years old.
She had surgery at 16 years old and had to stay in the hospital for 1 year for recovery because she was not healing.

It is common for people who come to see a homeopath to have seen a plethora of alternative practitioners before. This is especially true for the "2nd wave" people I discussed in Chapter 1.

She was given the homeopathic remedy *Phophorus* because she seems very outgoing and very chatty. In the broadest terms possible, these qualities might be indications for that remedy. The mistake here is that the homeopath didn't look at the disorder but rather looked at the personality. That is a big mistake.

At the moment of her first visit, she is taking a steroid-based medication.

Understanding the person's disorder on a very deep level is crucial. Previous remedies were not effective because while they matched some qualities of the case they

were constantly up and down, that's all I know."

Tell about your symptoms, please.

"My symptoms are loss of appetite, losing weight, nausea, diarrhea, constipation, bloatedness, blood in the stool, feeling lethargic and sleeping a lot. I have developed a fear of surgery and I am certain there must be a way to heal this area."

How does the Crohn's affect you, please?

"I think I am an overachiever and the Crohn's gets in the way. It's an obstacle and I get really panicked because of it. I just hope this is not going to lead to surgery. It brings me back to when I was 17 years old feeling like I let people down. I feel like someone gives me an opportunity to not do something when I am sick and I don't like that. There is a block here and I don't like it because I want to do what I want to do, so I ignore the pain but then I get sick even more."

Tell me about letting people down, please.

"I don't want people around when I am sick. "Just leave me alone." I get skinny and I don't like it. I see it as being sick; I don't see it as glamorous. I would love to do things, especially travel. I always want to be on the move and get a step up. Sales is stressful and it is not good for me but it gives me an opportunity

didn't match the core characteristics in the inner state. It is easy to give a remedy but it is not easy to give the correct one. Each case presents many different aspects and each one needs to be understood at its lowest common denominator. They need to be understood at the root that ties all complaints together. Only then can the proper remedy be given.

All the symptoms she is listing are common in Crohn's disease. They are good to know yet for the purpose of recommending a homeopathic remedy they are not very useful to find the best most accurate, individualized remedy.

There are a lot of leads here to ask a question: "overachiever, obstacle, panicked, back to 17, opportunity, blocked..." Any of these could probably tell us more. I chose the theme of "letting people down" because it seems attached to her youth. Generally, when people trace back to a young age the mind is less adulterated than it is later in

to shine, then the Crohn's stops me and that feels like a crutch."

Could you please tell me a little more about the feeling of a crutch, please?

"Everything else is not important. All the focus is on me getting better. I want to be surrounded by things that make me feel better, happy and make me laugh. I don't want to have to put on a show for anything or anybody."

Tell me the opposite feeling of that, please.

"It is the opposite of happy. It is knots in the stomach. I don't feel confident I feel self-guarded. I don't want to show anything. I let as little as possible out. I don't tell people about my fears and I fake being happy so that people don't worry. It feels like I let somebody down or that I don't live up to the standards. I feel totally empty and I think I'll make it up to you. When I get like this it seems as if I am not living up to what I promised. I am always happy-go-lucky but now I can't go 110. I can't deliver in relationship, job etc. I bend over with cramps and I get stiff with pain. I don't want people to see me on my low. I'm not giggly, I don't laugh, I am not happy, that's all."

Please don't stop talking, you are doing great. Continue to describe that state.

"I don't want to let something make me feel sad or angry. It is an empty feeling, I'm not laughing anymore. I can lash out in these moments. I hate people who are miserable. I

life and the answers to my questions are much easier to express.

When she says, "I don't want to have to put on a show," this makes me think of what she says about sales: "It gives me an opportunity to shine." It seems very show-or per-formance-like. The skill of the homeopath is not to lead the person down a certain path, but rather to remain centered and unprejudiced as to the direction of the case and to listen. This is the key. Thank heavens I didn't lead because the remedy was not at all part of the performance type of remedies we have.

get pain in my stomach. When I was younger my brother passed away and I thought that no one or anything can make me feel so bad."

Tell more about feeling empty, please.

"Empty means may be I should start a business but I am unproductive. Everybody has to do something. What have you done lately? I want to feel productive, otherwise I feel empty. Empty is the center of me. I am not strong and I can just break like this (motion as if she were breaking a stick). I can't do any of what I said before because I am weak and could break at any moment."

REMEDY:

Pix liquida

FOLLOW-UP:

Pierre: How have you been, please?

"So far so good. I have not had any intense pain on the right side. I am still taking Prednisone and Imuran but at a lower dose. I am also sleeping much better. The stress level is the same and I am able to handle it pretty well, even when things get chaotic. I don't feel any cramping in the stomach. The empty feeling I talked about is also not as strong."

What else can you tell me about the way you feel?

"I saw a black cat in my dream. I dreamt about my cat being sick, skinny and curled up in a

There comes a point when people need to use their hands in order to facilitate themselves in the expression of disorder. This level represents the meeting point or the root of the PEM. At this level the person is literally bringing the disorder alive for me. It is absolutely crucial to reach that point during the consultation. This is the deepest and the most individualizing level.

The physical symptoms for Crohn's are the same for most people but at this level the overlap disappears and individuality in disorder is revealed. The hand gesture puts the whole condition in motion and gives it life, which is what we are interested in. Recently someone was describing to me the feeling of falling and she was sitting motionless with her arms crossed on her chest. The words were coming out but they were not describing the feeling or the experience of falling. Until the body puts in motion the experience of falling, then there's no way to know what the remedy is.

ball. I just saw the back of his head and it was little. He lost a lot of weight and I felt sorry for this thing. It seemed almost as though it wanted to be like that. It was not eating right. I felt it was helpless and I just watched it. I can see myself in the same position as the cat and then it went away. When I saw it like that I felt I wanted to ask questions: 'What is it that you want to tell me?' and I felt somewhat cool but friendly."

REMEDY:

Continue.

FOLLOW UP:

Pierre: Are you as well as you were last month?

"I have stopped Prednisone completely after speaking with my doctor. I was only taking 2.5mg anyway. I am still taking Imuran 100mg. I can handle things in everyday life much better. Now, with hindsight, I see there has been a big difference, I am able to put things in perspective. I am sleeping better. Sleep is so sweet. I am feeling good so the last thing I think I am concerned with is being down. Productivity is very important to me and now that I feel good, it is really great to see good results. The cramping in the stomach is still much better and I didn't have any PMS symptoms."

REMEDY:

Continue

This Crohn's case may remind you of Launa's case of post-partum depression. There is a similarity. Indeed, the remedy is from the same family.

Astonishing! She dreams of a black cat and the cat is feeling exactly the way she is and she recognizes it as such. As a similar reflection of oneself, the dream itself becomes healing.

At this point she has improved dramatically and the best thing to do is continue on the same course and stay with the same remedy.

Naturally, I always encourage people to speak with their attending physician regarding any matter of medication much as I did in Mat's cardiac case. It is absolutely not my place to make any suggestions towards that matter at all. PMS is something most women don't mention during the first visit but once they notice that even that is better, then they think, "Wow! What else can you do?" Lali's case (see case) shows that you don't have to live with PMS.

After several years she continues to be well. For the long run she decided to remain on a non-therapeutic dose of Imuran "just in case" she has a flare-up. Perhaps, she could do without but her choice is the best for her. There is no point in my being dogmatic.

RUDY

(7 yr old)

MC: DYSLEXIA

- ADHD
- Double hernia at 1 yr old
- Tongue-tied
- Grinds his teeth at night
- Night terrors
- Anxiety around homework time

Pierre: Please tell me what brings you here.

Mother: "We have a big problem. I thought he was doing really well but since March he has not done well in school. He just can't sit still. In 1st grade it was really difficult for him. He likes to curse and destroy things. He fights with his sister a lot. He is also quite jealous and he tries to hurt her."

Tell me more about that, please.

"He is very disruptive. He has to know that he's going to win every time there is an argument about anything. You would think he would like sports but he doesn't participate in sports whatsoever. He really has a lot of trouble dealing with other boys, but on the other hand he is usually very affectionate with girls. "

I would like to know more about him. What could you tell me that is unusual about him, please?

DISCUSSION

Rudy has been receiving biofeedback for the last 3 months a couple of times a week.

I present this case to suggest that homeopathy could be tried early in the developmental stage of these conditions to "nip'em in the bud." Instead of medicating for the long term a child can be transformed from a hellish, difficult life to having a healthy, happy vibrant existence.

I noticed parents bring children with ADD or ADHD at the last minute. Usually the school has been asking for the child to be on medication for quite some time because they tend to be disruptive in class. The parents resist the pressure to medicate and they come in, after having tried everything they could think of, almost in a state of panic. Something must be done *now*. These are complex issues and to work under the gun is not comfortable. I hope this book can help bring children earlier into the homeopath's consultation room.

"He has very bad nightmares, night terrors actually. They are very scary with heads chopped off, giant rats with red glowing eyes, roaches and bees. He is petrified that someone is going to come in at night. Every night he makes sure that the alarm is on. He sleeps with the covers over his head and now he wants the light on at night. He is very, very scared. He also sweats a lot at night. He wakes up screaming at the top of his lungs. He is clearly scared of somebody or something. We can't understand what he says, he is so scared."

At this point, I was rather fascinated because the parent had not mentioned the dyslexia. Actually the dyslexia in this case was never mentioned nor explained but it was dealt with perfectly in the end, as we'll see.

That's very interesting. What else can you tell me?

"He says he is scared of dying. There is always this death stuff. He wants to know that his heart is beating. At night, he always calls out for his father as if he were being shot or hurt badly. The nights are really terrible. He also bangs his head against the wall at times which is very difficult to watch. We can't even stop him at times."

At night, he calls out for his father instead of his mother. It is a matter of life or death, it is not a nurturing issue in which case he would be asking for his mother.

It sounds like the pregnancy was very difficult and I assumed that the state of the child was similar to the mother's. The mother was terrified and so is he. Now I would not just assume it to be the case, I would take the case through the mother.

How was the pregnancy?

It was very difficult, I found out that I had placenta previa and I was petrified."

REMEDY:

Stramonium

At the time of this case, which was 15 years ago, I cross-referenced a few of his characteristic features and voila! The good old-fashioned way and it worked wonderfully. Do compare this case with

FOLLOW UP: (1 month)

Pierre: Is Rudy better?

Mother: "I would say so. He is not as annoyed by little things as he used to be before. I would say there is a major difference at night; he is not as scared. He doesn't even check the alarm or the door before going to sleep. He is not waking up screaming at the top of his lungs asking for his father. We can't thank you enough for the sleep we have been able to get. If he wakes up, he just calls out. It does not seem like he is getting nightmares anymore."

That's good to hear. Please tell me more.

"His anger is a lot better. He is not destroying things. He has not said, "I am really angry." He has not been disruptive in class. I don't think it has been bad I because his teacher has not called me. This is a big relief; we thought we would have to take him out of the school."

Is there anything that has not improved? What about the dyslexia?

"He still does not have interest in his homework or reading. It doesn't seem to interest him but as far as the dyslexia we have not noticed anything and his teachers have not said anything. If they don't say anything, we are not going to raise the issue."

REMEDY:

Continue

Erika's lupus case for example. The level of details is vastly different. It is like watching a black white TV and then switching to color. In Erika's case, one can actually feel the way she is. Here we only have an idea, which, fortunately, was good enough to recommend something accurate.
Comparing these two cases really shows the reason why we are so much more accurate now than back then a few years ago.

The main issue was presented as dyslexia, but I think ADHD was their biggest concern. In the end, the ADHD and the dyslexia (and much more) were resolved. That is the way homeopathy works.

Can you imagine how much more peaceful the house must be now and how much rest everyone is getting? The whole family is affected when a child is struggling like this. It is not the child's fault of course; it is the disorder that is making life like that.

"He doesn't have the internal violence ha had before." I find that statement so very

SEVERAL FOLLOW-UPS: (The remedy was repeated a few times)

Mother: "He continues to be good. He doesn't have that internal violence he had before. He was always a good kid, but looking back he was so scared. School is easier, as well as the time doing his homework. He is not first of his class, but he is fine."

revealing. The way she says it is like something has been removed from the child. It is not the same as saying "He is OK, he is less disruptive." "The internal violence has been removed. That is deep and beautiful. There is so much less emotional pain.

I think "internal violence" is an interesting way of putting it. The mother's sense is that his interior nature is better. This is very substantive, astute and insightful.

VALERIE

(Late 20's)

DISCUSSION

MC: HORMONAL IMBALANCE DUE

TO MISCARRIAGE

- Two miscarriages
- Allergies

The miscarriage was caused by a molar pregnancy, which is an abnormality of the placenta, caused by a genetic error during the fertilization of the egg. Molar pregnancies are rare, occurring in 1 out of every 1,000 pregnancies. There are two types of molar pregnancies, "complete" and "partial."

Pierre: Please, tell me what is troubling you?

"I had two miscarriages in the last eight months and my hormones are not returning back to normal levels. When I was 25 years old, I had a polyp on the uterus removed. I bled for three months and I wonder if it has anything to do with my problem now although I should tell you that I don't think so since I already have a child and I didn't have any problems with that pregnancy."

I can't comment on the medical part, but do ask your doctor about it. Tell me more, please.

"I have allergies as well with some pain on the bridge of my nose. It got worse when I started working as a computer operator. I quit work and my allergies got better, but up to this day my nose still itches and runs in the morning."

She suffered a miscarriage several months before and she is quite concerned about her hormonal levels not returning back to normal levels. Yet, she mentions her allergies. I love it. It has to do with the fact that we ask open-ended questions, which make people feel at ease to talk about anything that troubles them.

OK, what else?

"I have been spotting since my last miscarriage. The flow has not completely shut down. There

Now she is back to more important issues. It doesn't mean that allergies are not important, but at this point they are a little secondary.

is substantial spotting after intercourse, which is like menstruating for one day then some pinkish stuff remains. I also have a discharge, cottage cheese type with brown discoloration. My doctor tells me my hormone levels have still not come down, they should be down because it has been six months since I've had the miscarriage."

Tell me more about how you have been since the miscarriage, please.

"Ever since the miscarriage, I have been tired. I am exhausted all the time. I have tingling in my arms and legs but not in the muscles. Instead I feel some tingling in my veins as if they have been pulled. All of a sudden, I realized I have veins from the elbow and down my arms. I also have some pain around my right and left wrist right in between the bones."

Tell me more about the pain in your veins, please.

"They feel pulled and then there is rest. They feel stretched out and I feel the aftermath of it. All the network of my veins hurts at the same time. There is a little buzzing in the veins. I want to be stretched; I want someone to pull my body out. It feels as if there are bubbles in between them. I also have the same feeling in my wrists and ankles, as if there are air bubbles. I am not sure what else I can tell you."

A strange, rare or peculiar symptom is always relevant in homeopathy. "Tingling in the veins" or "as if they were pulled" is such a symptom. Valerie is very expressive and she gives a beautiful, vivid description of her physical pains. The more details she gives, the more clues are brought to the fore about the remedy.

"I am not sure what else I can tell you." Not knowing what to say is very common as I explained in Dana's case of IBS. Most people feel like they have little or no more to say, and yet I ask another question and I get a little more information which propels us forward. This is not easy - although it may appear so from these cases - but keep in mind they are edited.

She says, "doing a simple task feels like a lot," which is contradictory to "feeling better after a work out," therefore for my purpose of finding a

Please don't stop, it is very interesting for me.

"The feet and the hands are usually not affected. I can't do anything. I can't even put my son to bed. I just lie there and go to sleep myself. One of the problems is that I still feel tired after I wake up. I have been exhausted for some time now. For some reason, I feel better after I work out. Before my last miscarriage I had become a vegan but now I really feel tired throughout the day. I don't know if it has anything to do with it all."

remedy it is interesting. Again we are looking at SRP's.

The description of her symptoms related exactly to the experience of diver's sickness called "the bends." Bubbles form in the body when the body is not allowed to decompress properly from being deep under water. The remedy she needs is clear to me.

REMEDY:

Nitrogen

FOLLOW UP:

Pierre: Are you feeling better?

"I am well. I don't feel tired anymore. I always needed coffee to get me alive and awake. Now I get up at 7 a.m. and I feel great."

That's good. Please tell me more.

"I forgot to tell you the last time but I used to have nausea and some dizziness, both have been much better. The air bubbles are gone. My hormones levels are down. I can tell you now that I felt like I was in a deep dark place. I preferred hiding somewhere in the dark, away from people. During this past month I remembered I had this feeling of bubbles in

With hindsight she realized how "deep of a place" she was in. This is an interesting choice of words very much relating to the diver similarity I mentioned before.
Also with hindsight more memories are coming back to her. As her health is coming back, the retracing of the VF (Vital Force) is bringing up memories. It is a good thing because it brings more consciousness and that is always better than carrying hidden material.

my veins many times before, particularly after doing something strenuous."

Isn't it interesting how things come back to your mind when you are looking back?

"I've always liked to have a little bit of pain, a little soreness; I stretch and I feel the parts alive. It's alive because I can feel the pain. That part of my body exists. I like the soreness of a little cut. Even as a child I remember liking it. The only pain I ever wanted to get rid of was labor pain. I didn't like the whole commotion of the hospital. They were rushing in and out I could not relax. I was happy it was all over."

The homeopathic remedy *Nitrogen* relates to the childbirth's stage of the final release of the child and letting it come out. The hormones released during delivery naturally stop as the process comes to an end. In this case, because of her general state, they never stopped the release, as the body was not recognizing that the pregnancy was over.

She continues to be very well.

DANNA

(Early 40's)

MC: H PYLORI

IBS

- GI tract
- History of gallstones
- Chronic yeast infection
- Spider veins
- Severe PMS

Pierre: Please tell me what is going on?

"I have PMS with bloating. I get very moody and irritable and I feel like I am on the warpath."

OK, what else is going on?

"I have allergies in the spring from March to April. I get an itchy nose and I sneeze a lot."

What else?

"I have pretty severe spiders veins that are painful if I sit down for a long time. When I sit, the pain starts behind the knee and it gets much worse during the summer."

What else?

"I have very painful intercourse and I also have chronic yeast infection."

What else?

"I have hemorrhoids."

DISCUSSION

This case is presented because it is elucidated through her dreams. In homeopathy, we are not really interested in the dream itself as that can be open to interpretation.

Open any book on dreams and you will quickly notice wide differences in what an elephant in a dream might mean. As a homeopath, I am interested in the feelings in the dream. At the root, the dreams always match the emotional and mental level and show what is going on deeply in the constitutional disorder. George's case of ADHD is a great example of that. In this case, the dream combined with other symptoms made the remedy very clear to me.

Within the first sentence she talks about being on the "warpath" the tone is set!

It is common for people to speak for 15 minutes non-stop. I generally have a hard time keeping up with the writing as things are being rattled off in quick-fire style. It is also common for people to stop after one or two sentences and wait for me to ask a question; it is so in this case.

When people struggle with the questions, I often hear, "I can't tell you anymore than that," Or, "That's it, I

I think when we spoke on the phone you mentioned IBS (Irritable Bowel Syndrome)?

"Yes. I can't eat. I have heartburn and most of the time I have gas no matter what I eat or drink. These problems have progressively gotten worse over the last ten years. I never really drank orange juice when I first came to this country, but now I really can't drink it as I get major burning in my throat if I do."

Describe the symptoms to me a little more, please.

"Even when I drink water I belch. I call it an empty belch. For me it is so strange that without eating I belch. I always blame my diet of sweets. The whole thing is definitely worse when I eat chocolate or anything creamy. Everything is worse when I eat meat but I also can't eat fruits or vegetables such as broccoli, cabbage."

Please continue.

" I get diarrhea as soon as I drink coffee and the same is true if I eat any citrus. I felt better after I cut milk. If I drink milk, I feel like there is a net in my throat and food gets caught there. I feel like the throat needs to expand to let the food pass. I try to swallow but my stomach is pushing everything back up. I choose very tiny pieces to swallow and I never eat a big piece of meat."

I am sure there is a lot more you can tell me. Please continue.

"I get severe heartburn and reflux. I have burning in the throat. It all comes up in my can't say more." The initial consultation can be difficult for these people as they feel they have little to say. Truth be told, there is always more to say, really.

Here so far we are only building a list of complaints. When this happens I often stop asking questions and I explain why I am asking them. Most of the time it breaks the ice and then it all unfolds very nicely.

Not being able to eat most foods is very common for people suffering of IBS. Many alternative practitioners commonly recommend a restricted diet because they blame candida in the G.I. tract and attempt at getting rid of it with diet and detoxification of the colon. I have seen this help sometimes as long as the person stays on the diet, but then after a while the symptoms come back at which point further restrictions are needed. This is a classic case of a dog chasing its own tail; it doesn't lead anywhere in the long run. Foods can provide some relief if the condition is minor. I talk a little more about diet in Celeste's case of IBS. While we should be mindful of the food we eat, blaming it for our problems is really misleading.

Others think antibiotics wreak havoc with the intestinal flora. At last count, there are over 350 different types

throat. I started paying attention to it 20 years ago. I eat something and that's it, it starts. As soon as I eat something, I feel bloated and the colon feels like it is pushing. I get the urge to go to bathroom. The gas is really horrible. My system is in rebellion with what I eat. I get very loud rumbling noises in the abdomen and I feel like there is pushing in the rectum. It is as if there is something broken and the system cannot handle it. It is like everything is falling apart and then there is one big pain. I feel so sick I cannot function. I feel depressed, nervous and anxious. I can't handle it, and I can't control the craving; it is stronger than I am. I just have to accept it. I feel so miserable and helpless that there is something stronger. I have accepted it. I am very suspicious and careful. Just because everything is fine this minute does not mean something is not going to happen the next."

I get the sense that you want to tell me something, please tell me what is on your mind.

"I love chocolate. I need to have it. I love the smell of it and the taste of it. It satisfies my hunger for sweets. I can't help it. I have to have it. As soon as I eat something sweet everything is all right. It hits the spot (pointing below her ribs) and I can go about my life. I feel satisfied, happy, yet at the same time I feel guilty because I may be creating the problem. It can destroy your health, you know. I can't have one piece of chocolate. I have to have

of bacteria in the intestines. I have even heard that between 50 to 75% of our body weight may be bacteria. If this is true (and there is no reason to believe that it is not), can we even begin to know what antibiotics have done to our overall body ecology and what they have caused in the long run? Thank heavens this doesn't have anything to do with homeopathy.

"It is stronger than I am and I accept it" is the coping mechanism. Understanding the speed of the case is a crucial part of the initial consultation. For example, in Clara's case of lupus there is total destruction, and in Tom's case of migraines it is an attack and then there is relief. The cases in this book give all of the different possibilities so far identified.

Outside of homeopathy one would say, "You need to overcome this desire of having to have chocolate." This is such a harsh thing to say - and you chocolate lovers know what mean! She is aware of that but she can't. She says it when she states, "It is stronger than I am." In any case, I doubt it would make a difference.

Freedom is what homeopathy is all about on the physical, emotional and mental level. In this case, the result for her should be to be able

the whole thing. I can't only have one cookie, I have to have a whole bunch. I definitely have something missing."

Tell me more about that please.

"It is something that is coming from the inside. The stomach has a sucking sensation. Something needs to be fed and I get so hungry that I have to feed it. On the other hand, fish smell and taste makes me nauseous. Even the ocean smell is not acceptable to me. Even passing by a seafood store triggers the nausea. The smell is atrocious for me. I don't know what to tell you anymore."

Talk to me about the warpath?

"It started as a teenager. I am Dr. Jekyll and Mr. Hyde. Seven days before my periods I get really upset and I want to quarrel with people. I can't control that. It is stronger than I am. I get severe cravings for sweets. I get mad and upset at everybody. Just look at me the wrong way and I am ready to fight. It is like striking a match, but I cannot control it. It happens so suddenly it always amazes me. Everything is stronger. It's like politics; I cannot control it so I'd rather not listen to anything."

Please describe the feeling of having something stronger than you.

"It makes me feel helpless, upset and angry. I cannot take over and change it."

to have chocolate without having such a need for it. She should no longer suffer from IBS and H. pylori. Yes, it is possible!

I was so steeped in her delightful chocolate craving, imagining smooth, silky buttery taste in my mouth that the contrast she made with the fish was nauseating to me, too.

Now that she has told me her guilt or her sin about the chocolate, she feels she has nothing left to say and I should be able to figure this out but I need to have more information so I go back to something I don't understand in the context of the totality of symptoms. I ask her about "the warpath."

She wants to quarrel before her period. She doesn't want to but "it is stronger." This is the same feeling as when she was speaking of chocolate. It is also how she spoke of her IBS pains and politics. Now we are seeing that problem from four different issues. All around, it is the same perception. We are getting closer to the root of it *all*. The whole disorder can be nailed.

I am trying different ways to get to the root level and I am still missing relevant information to make a good choice of remedy. She is still reluctant to give me information.

Tell me about your dreams. Any dream that had a particular impression on you or any recurrent dream in your lifetime.

"I am in an area with a lot of trees. I don't like desert at all. This place is calm and beautiful. The trees are tall with a lot of branches and very green. That's why I like a real Christmas trees. I would hug the trees. I have this strange sensation as if I belong with the trees. I should be there. I feel safe with them. I need them for my survival. I am feeling calm, carefree and happy with them. Without them I feel weak rather than strong. It is like the IBS. It makes me feel as if I can break at any time like a tree branch. I could just break in two. I could just snap."

REMEDY:

Sabina

FOLLOW UP:

Pierre: How have you been feeling?

"I used to have nausea all the time. Now it is not nearly as bad as it used to be. It was especially bad in the morning but I must say that it is a lot better. I have also noticed that my PMS has been better as well. This time I didn't even get cramps. I had a yeast infection after taking the remedy but it went away on its own."

Did anything else get better?

"The throat feels normal now. Not tight or constricted and when I swallow I don't feel

I change the approach with the hope of getting the information in a different way. I decide to go the dreams route. Often, they give me the opening I need to get deeper. To the homeopath the dreams are an integral part of understanding the case. It is not something outside the person that needs to be interpreted. The dreams are used as an extension of life. They are connected to the waking state just like the physical level is connected to the emotional and mental level. There is no break in the continuum. It can't be any other way.

As she says, "I could break in two," she spontaneously makes a gesture as if she were breaking a stick. Now that she has put life into the case, she is using all of her senses to express the disorder.

Now she can go to a party and eat everything but in lesser quantity. This is good but it is not the time to indulge in food. It is understandable that she would eat more from time to time after several years of guilt about eating food. This reminds me of a woman who was re-

like I am going to choke. Three days ago I had the feeling that it was getting narrow again.

Last week at a party I ate everything but not as much as I normally would and I had some symptoms but they went away quickly. Before, I would have felt really terrible and the symptoms would have been really bad."

How is the craving for chocolate?

"The craving of chocolate is strong if I see it, whereas before I had to have it. I would not even think about it, I had to have it. The feeling of something missing is not as bad. The craving I had there (pointing under the ribs) is not as strong anymore. The feeling that something needs to be fed is much better. It is really not as strong."

Tell me more about the IBS, please.

"I still get some rumbling, but I am much better. I have some bloating and some urge to go to the bathroom but overall that is also much better. The gas has improved as well. I don't feel as bad, I don't feel as if I am going to break or as if something is broken. My whole system is working. I feel like it is under control. It is not stronger than I am. I was depressed before. I wouldn't acknowledge it, but now I don't see things in such dark colors. I don't get as scared about food any more. If I don't have such a good day I look at it now that tomorrow will be better."

ally seriously debilitated by migraines and since she was feeling much better she figured she would catch up on socializing with friends and family. I am thrilled she is so much better but I advised to slow down a bit. She said to me that she didn't know how long the relief would last and that she wanted to take advantage of it. She continues to be well, took a step back and a great life is unfolding.

Now that health is being restored, everything is getting easier and look at that chocolate craving. She needs much less of it. It is no longer a craving like it was before. The reason for that is that her inner state is far healthier.

REMEDY:

Continue

SEVERAL FOLLOW-UPS:

"I am especially happy that I don't have to go to the bathroom after eating. I also got ill only once this winter whereas it used to be several times. The PMS is so much better now. I have been better. No nausea. G.I: Empty belch is far better. The feeling that something needs to be fed is much better. The feeling that something is broken is almost gone."

CELESTE

(Early 30's)

MC: Irritable Bowel Syndrome (IBS)

- H-Pylori
- Cold sores
- Vertigo

Pierre: Please tell me what brings you here?

"I used to have a cast-iron stomach. I never had any difficulties digesting anything until I went to a social event after which I had diarrhea for a week-and-a-half. I took an antibiotic for it. I was okay for a couple of years and then my stomach started to feel bloated and I got constipated. Then I got diarrhea, abdominal pain and the vomiting started. I ended up losing five pounds. I had the feeling of an air pocket in my stomach with severe gas and heartburn. They checked me for everything even celiac disease as I was sure I had it."

Please continue.

"By 11 a.m. I have a very ravenous appetite. I get so hungry but then I eat one cracker and I have pain right in the middle of my ribs. I've been belching after eating for the last nine years. I can't even sleep well. I have so much less energy, I hardly go to the gym and I certainly don't want to go out to eat. I go back and forth between constipation and diarrhea, which is at least five times a day. I get a sudden desire to go to the bathroom and it can be explosive. As soon as I get cramps in

DISCUSSION

IBS and H pylori have become very common. Some claim that it is a result of over-prescribing antibiotics and killing gastro intestinal bacteria indiscriminately. That is a debate I don't get into. My only purpose is to do something about the whole problem without adhering to a theory or a cause.

I present this case because even with not enough follow-up visits much could be done. This situation happens when people don't know enough about homeopathy and decide that as symptoms have cleared that's enough for them. I disagree with that because health can be restored at far deeper levels and can be an incredible investment in one's person.

I think there is a detail we should all keep in mind: a lot of food preparation in this country is simply not hygienic enough and causes enormous problems to a lot of people. Be very judicious of where you eat.

So far, the symptoms she has detailed - diarrhea, abdominal pain, etc. - are common to the IBS condition.

my stomach I have to go. Medication has not helped. I hear some rumbling immediately after eating. I start to sweat profusely and I change my shirt several times within a couple of hours. The pain is so bad I am hunched over. Symptoms start with belching, and then I feel bloating, which is followed by gas. Gas smells as if something died, something festering. It even lingers in the room for a long time. I can't stay in the living room I have to stay in another room it is so bad. The air pocket in the stomach feels like pressure. There is fullness and hunger at the same time. It feels as if I'm going to explode. All of my symptoms feel much worse in the evening. It is extremely uncomfortable. I can't be near anybody with this. It feels as if someone old should have this."

She is still giving symptoms that are rather common to IBS. It doesn't mean they are not important to know, but up to now there are few SRP's so nothing is really individualizing the condition.

Please, tell me about the pain.

"The pain just comes on after eating. The gas is extremely unpleasant and offensive. I certainly wouldn't want my wife to have this but I have it. I have broken down and cried. It is zapping my energy, it's constricting. When I was young, I was overweight. I was teased for being overweight and right now I would be happy eating a whole pie and not having symptoms. I have restricted my diet so much. Bloating is always difficult. I don't want to deal with this any longer."

She describes the odor as "offensive." The pain is "constricting." Now it is becoming an individualizing and vivid description of what is going on. From my point of view, it is really wonderful to hear. And now she is still going back to when she was overweight. I would have loved to have more feelings but that's all I could get. As I mentioned, it is a very deep case like most of the cases here, but it demonstrates that even half way down the root relief can happen.

When we talk about IBS or any other gastro intestinal problems, we have to talk about diet because many people think it is related.

REMEDY:

Carbo vegetabilis

FOLLOW UP:

Pierre: Please tell me how you are?

"The air pocket is much better. The heartburn, belching, diarrhea, sleep, most of the symptoms I had are no longer a major issue. I still have some gas and bloating but not everyday."

SEVERAL FOLLOW-UPS LATER:

Pierre: How have you been?

"Great. During vacation, I had many frozen drinks and I felt okay. I have some slight distension. I am definitely not as bad as when first started. I am feeling the light at the end of the tunnel. I don't have the explosive diarrhea, I am more regular and I gained 4 pounds. Having dinner with the family is much more enjoyable. I am able to sit down in the living room with my family."

COMMENT:

One last word about food. As much as we can, we should eat organic, fresh food that is not processed. Eating processed food is like putting faulty fuel in your car. Food is meant to be physically nutritious with vitamins, proteins, minerals and lipids. It should also be as emotionally satisfying as possible.

I do have a couple of things to say more particularly about restricted diet. In my experience:

1: Unless one is extremely regimented, it is not possible to stay on such a diet for any extended period of time;

2: The first thing we do in life is eat. Then every day of our lives we eat several times a day. At a minimum, it is extremely important!

3: It really exacerbates me to see diets that don't address the emotional aspect of food. To me cutting a food out or, worse, a whole food group such as carbohydrates, is as bad emotionally as it is nutritionally. It is also not sustainable in the long run.

The only diet worth following is eating less food than you are eating now. Feeling hungry is actually a good thing. We don't have to feed the body with food - much like an addict feeds the habit - every time we are hungry. Drink a glass of water instead especially at night.

After all these years she is feeling better! Frozen drinks and no diarrhea. Those were a big no-no before. Here's life. Who am I to say she shouldn't have a margarita. These are good results, yet more could be done. The Vital Force does wonders and for it to restore the whole digestive tract takes a long time nowadays.

GAYA

(Early 40's)

MC: INSOMNIA

• Fatigue

• Muscle soreness

Pierre: Please tell me what troubles you?

"I have lost a huge amount of stamina. I can't exert myself nearly the same way I used to be able to: I can't exercise and I am increasingly getting worse. Early in 2001, at the height of my physical health, I was in the best shape I could be in and going to yoga several times a week. On the day following each yoga class, I would be so sore that I eventually stopped going. I felt I was doing myself more harm than good. Now, I get tired just walking 20 blocks. Even sex is hard to recover from. It calms the psyche but physically it does not feel good, especially the day after. When I exercise it feels good, it's afterward that I have problems. My big fear with these two problems is that I am headed for some destiny. My father has MS. He is not a happy man; he never was. I am not like that but the MS really scares me. I hate to say it, but I am predisposed to it."

Please continue. This is all very interesting to me.

"In 2004, I remember having to travel and I was taking melatonin, so perhaps it started around that time. Now I take Ambien. I started a relationship around this time and it was a

DISCUSSION

I present this case for everyone who suffers from insomnia. I have noticed puzzlement in insomniacs. The feeling is like "How can I not sleep? It is as natural as eating or being awake and yet it is not happening. What's wrong with me?" The frustration is great and the fatigue is even greater. Sometimes a lack of understanding can be compounded by friends who might regard insomnia as a psychosomatic problem and say, "Just relax." It is a difficult ailment for people to grasp and have sympathy.

difficult adjustment. I was staying up late and messing up my sleep regimen and something triggered that keeps me up at night now. So far, the only thing that has made a difference is magnesium citrate powder."

Tell me more about the insomnia, please.

"My mother passed away and that was a major life event. It is the biggest thing that has happened to me. Thinking about that event puts me back in a really bad place. I started to hear my heart while falling asleep. There are nights when I don't sleep at all. I am so exhausted all the time. Some nights I only sleep one or two hours."

How is the insomnia affecting you?

"I feel I've lost enthusiasm. I avoid social situations because I am too tired. I find there is such a correlation between the insomnia and my relationship. There is also this fear of being like my father, of not being able to work because it is so bad."

Could you tell me about the correlation with your relationship, please?

"When this relationship started, my boyfriend was holding back a lot and it was upsetting to me. He constantly sent me mixed signals that lead me be apprehensive about our relationship. I had to wonder. I am so susceptible to this kind of anxiety. The insomnia started around the time that my

She says sleep with Ambien does not feel like real sleep. "The eyes are closed, but it is not the same thing as real sleep."

I say, "Tell me more about the insomnia," and her answer is about her mother. It is the sufferer who weaves the whole tapestry of the condition on all levels. My purpose is to listen and go where she leads me. Using her words, I probe further and further until we reach the very root of what ties everything together. I picture this process like two happy kids running in a field of wheat: the sun is warm and we are walking back home but the wheat is taller than us, so we are going blind trying to pick up clues as to where we stand. Then we reach the edge of the field and I know exactly where we are. This is the way I see the process of finding the remedy. Sometimes I try to take a shortcut, which is like jumping up to see over the wheat. Rarely do the shortcuts get me anywhere.

If you feel this process is radically different from medicine, I would say that you are right. In fact, it is the exact opposite. To me the person with

mother received some horrible news about our family. I remember in a flat second that nothing was going to be the same with my family."

Continue please. Tell me more.

"The day my mother died, I knew it would send me into orbit. Family for me is a core and I say that because I don't have one of my own. Being without one... Oh, gosh. It's petrifying to think about it."

Tell me more about family, please.

"I lived in a foreign country for a while. The newness of it was great, but I found that others don't know you on the inside. This is you and then there is this whole other thing; you can never feel you are "in" because they don't know all the history, all the details of growing up together. Without my mother I feel isolated. With her I always knew there was an unmitigated, unconditional feeling that she would understand and care for me. You can only get that from family."

It's wonderful to have had that. Please tell me more.

"None of my relationships have worked out. I was uprooted four times and I didn't have friends. I need to be in a relationship, but when I am in a relationship I feel very self-conscious. I have such a difficult time asking for basic needs. I can't just snap it off. Without

the **problem knows more than anybody else. Part of my job is to bring it all out to the point where it all comes together for the purpose of giving a remedy that matches.**

Correlating the insomnia with her relationship, her mother and her family appears as the central theme. As you read these cases you may find some themes seemingly obvious or simplistic. What is really important to understand is that she is telling me what she feels. No one else can know this. Together these themes form the gestalt that includes insomnia, fatigue and soreness.
Fatigue with insomnia can be rationalized. Most people who have insomnia are tired but soreness can't be rationalized since not all people suffering from insomnia get sore the way she does.

Inasmuch as the insomnia compels her to focus, it is the same feeling as when she is in a relationship and as when she was in Italy. In short, without a family she needs to focus because she "feels like an orphan." She does not

sleep I need to focus more, it is the same as with my relationship. It is the same as when I was in Italy. I feel the same way. I feel like I am an orphan. I just don't feel like I am part of anything or anybody."

REMEDY:

Magnesium carbonicum

FOLLOW-UP:

Pierre: How are you feeling, are you sleeping more?

"Within one to two days I felt different. Sleep within the last two weeks has been up and down, but when I don't sleep I don't have that feeling of panic anymore. The first two weeks were much better. Now it has been more difficult to fall asleep and stay asleep. Like I said, I don't feel panicked about it, I don't find myself obsessing about going to bed at a particular time like I did before, but it is not as good as it was a month ago when I started the remedy."

I am very happy to hear this, tell me more, please.

"My energy has been better. The muscle soreness is also a lot better. I have a stronger sense of being in my relationship than I did before. He seems so much more relaxed. I don't feel like it is a horrendous match."

feel part of a group. These are the opposite feelings to when she had her mother. The soreness after intimacy also relates to a relationship. Not being able to break away from a relationship is stating the obvious.

This case requires a remedy that has family as its central theme and the overall symptoms she suffers from. The homeopathic remedy will resolve all of her issues in a deep acting fashion upon the Vital Force.

In her case, the only thing that helps her a bit is magnesium citrate. A lot of insomniacs take it to sleep; it is palliative, which means that as long as you take it you don't have symptoms. As soon as you stop taking it, the symptoms come back. In homeopathy, magnesium relates to a family or group just like it is in this case. What was a little trickier to figure out in this case was the other half because magnesium can't be given by itself. I gave *Magnesium carbonicum* because of her feeling like an orphan as well as her affinity to her father's illness. There are many other choices available to the homeopath. Had the specificity been about the

Good. Could you tell me a little about hearing your heartbeat at night, please?

"For the first two weeks it was not beating heavily or racing like before, but it has been back in the last couple of weeks."

Have you had any dreams?

"My dreams have been in relation to my mother or father but they have been pleasant."

REMEDY:

Continue

SEVERAL FOLLOW-UPS LATER:

"I have discontinued Ambien. I am feeling well and paying attention to the things that can keep me from sleeping well. I mainly have good nights. I have been sleeping in hotels for the last couple of months because of business and that's been great. The muscle soreness and fatigue are just about gone too."

brother the remedy would have been *Magnesium phosphoricum*. Had it been about the mother, *Magnesium muriaticum* would have been appropriate.

The thing to do here is simply to continue. Everything is moving in the right direction.

The remedy was repeated several times through different follow-ups. She remains well.

ANNA

(Early teens)

DISCUSSION

MC: BILATERAL CHRONIC INFLAMMATION OF THE MIDDLE EARS WITH TYMPANIC PERFORATION
(Draining ears)
- Low physical stamina
- Pains in the legs
- Irritability

I present this case because this child went to see the best professors and heads of pediatric departments at famous NYC hospitals and they were stumped. A simple remedy resolved the whole problem and much more, gracefully, easily and without pain.

Pierre: Please, tell me as much as you can about these "draining ears."

Mother: "My daughter has had chronic ear infections for the last two years. The diagnosis from Mount Sinai Hospital says "very severe bilateral chronic inflammation with bilateral tympanic membrane perforations." She had a tonsillectomy and adenoidectomy a few years ago. She has very low physical stamina; she seems to always be dragging her feet. She always complains of stomach pains and various other abdominal problems. She gets high fevers of 104º F. She has cavities in her teeth and, last but not least, she always complains that her legs hurt."

This is a long name for the simple fact that her ears were in such bad shape that they were constantly oozing a yellowish liquid.

Antibiotics were prescribed numerous times weakening the Vital Force further.

Could you tell me more about the ear infections?

Mother: "She has a constant low grade fever which spikes at times. She spikes sudden fevers

She spikes 104ºF fevers. A severe reaction of this kind tells us that the Vital Force

162

of 104ºF, which get progressively worse at night. Her cheeks get flushed, her face turns red, and her eyes become glassy. She also gets very listless. When she was about two years old she stopped talking for a few months following a high fever. The ears drain yellowish brown liquid all the time. Yellowish liquid literally drips out of her ears all day, every day."

may be very strong, yet it should be so since she is only 12 years old.

We have two main remedies (and many more) for a fever that spikes or starts suddenly: *Belladonna* and *Ferrum phosphoricum*. If either one were given at the beginning of the fever the whole situation could be avoided.

Could you tell me more about Anna, more particularly when she is sick as well as her history, please?

Mother: "Up until she was six or seven years old she needed a stroller because she tires easily. Her eyes used to get very crusty and because of the enlargement of her tonsils she could hardly speak. She used to get into rages, responding to everything with anger. She had an inability to be calm. She has calmed down now but it doesn't take much to start her off, especially in the morning."

At a very young age Anna was already experiencing low stamina. Let's assume her ears could get "fixed." OK, great but what about the pain in her legs and not having energy? They are an integral part of the disorder.
The remedy can uproot the whole condition and free her of this encroachment upon her health setting up a return to health as a liberation of the PEM.

Tell me about being tired, please.

Anna: "My eyes hurt a little and sometimes I can't keep them open. I really don't have energy to walk. My legs hurt and then I get very cold. It feels like someone hit my legs."

Please, tell more.

Anna: "I have not slept through the night since I was seven or eight years old. I get up at least two or three times a night. I wake up all freaked out from nightmares. This morning

The feeling "as if somebody is behind me or somebody is in the room" is a common feature of a certain kind of remedies. This is a facet of the case that gives a good clue

I thought somebody was coming in my room. In my dreams, I feel my hands start to get cold and I shiver. I start to get scared and my body starts to hurt like someone is smacking me. It feels the same as when my foot hurts. It stings like little pins and needles and then it feels as if a rock falls on it."

Mother: "She is particularly irritated when she wakes up. Nobody can tell her anything."

Could you tell me about the sensation of being smacked?

Anna: "It stings and it hurts. I don't like being touched. I don't like it when people come up to me either, because I don't know what to expect."

Is there anything else I should know?

Mother: "She almost never sweats. She just gets red and overcome by the heat, which can lead to an easy heat stroke."

REMEDY:

Senecio aureus

FOLLOW-UP: (one month later)

Pierre: What can you tell me? Any good news?

in the process of choosing a remedy.

She said before that her legs were "hurting as if someone hit my legs." Now we have the feeling of being smacked at night, the root sensation for all is the same. It must be around this feeling of being hit.

This is a perfect description for my purposes of giving the most accurate remedy. The plant family called compositae has this precise sensation of being physically hit as in a total invasion to boundaries. Now I need to find the right one within that group which the previous clue of sensing a presence gives me.

One could think that with such a description the child might be getting hit all the time. It could not be further from the truth. I even asked the question. There is no doubt this child is being brought up in a nonviolent household. Read on...

Anna: "My ears are not leaking like they used to. My stomach has been much better, it doesn't hurt anymore. I also had bumps on my arms which are gone now. I have much more energy. I have not been tired."

Mother: "She has not been complaining as much and the low-grade fever is gone."

Tell me how all this happened, how it unfolded.

Anna: "I am not as cranky in the morning when I wake up.

When the totality of the disorder fits the homeopathic remedy perfectly, the results can only be perfect.

The tingling in my legs, feet and hands has also gotten much better."

How about your dreams?

Anna: "I have not had any nightmares and I have been sleeping a lot better. About two weeks ago, I remembered a place called "Discovery Zone" where kids would hit you or touch you purposely like in the ball pool. I don't know why I remembered that. Maybe it's because I noticed that I don't mind being touched now as much as I minded before."

She is substantially better physically, the ears are fine and emotionally her moods are fabulously better, but she felt a presence this week. This is what I call a precursor. If nothing were to be done at this point, she would probably start having nightmares again and wake up cranky and physically feel like she has been hit. Then the ears would start draining again. That's the totality in this case. That's the "roll call" of symptoms in this case. Repeating at this time will boost her

Would you say you are continuing to get better, have stopped getting better, or have gotten worse lately?

Anna: "Just this week I felt a presence in the room. I had not felt that for a while. It had completely gone away for a while."

REMEDY:

Repeat

SEVERAL FOLLOW-UPS LATER:

Anna: "I have had lots of energy. The bumps on my arms are gone."
Mother: "She is not complaining, nor is she irritable. We are very happy."

THREE YEAR FOLLOW-UP:

She has been for the most part. Getting cranky for the last few weeks.

REMEDY

Repeat.

Vital Force again and set her at a higher level of health. If we wait to repeat then the Vital Force will weaken further. The remedy must be repeated until the Vital Force can sustain a healthy state.

CLARA

(Late 30's)

MC: LUPUS ERYTHROMATOSUS

• Hyperthyroid

Pierre: Please tell me about the lupus.

"The lupus started with pain in the joints of my hands, I can't even open them now. They felt numb. When I started taking medication for the lupus I developed a high fever of 104°F and decided I would prefer to stay away from the medication but in the end I couldn't because of the pain."

OK, continue please.

"When I get sick I get *freezing cold*. It feels as if I am going to die. It truly feels as if I were dying. This coldness has been with me for three years, it is like an ice cube and I shiver. It starts in the legs and it goes up my body. When it starts, I begin to shake violently from the coldness. At that moment, I need to be around people. I even start to babble like a baby during the cold."

Could you tell me about this coldness, please?

"The cold is like an attack. When it goes away I feel very weak. After the shaking stops I sweat and then the coldness stops. Then I develop a rash and after that I feel healthy again but

DISCUSSION

This lupus case gives a good contrast of the way we used to choose a remedy and the way we do it now (which I talk about throughout this book) all wrapped into one. As homeopathy has gone through a renaissance, knowledge and accuracy have improved immensely. The difference is as wide as the difference between a Ford Model T and a 2008 BMW. Today's consultation is a lot more fluid and precise albeit a little more challenging because the questions asked are much more insightful of the disorder.

Although she is taking steroid medication the symptoms of lupus are acting up. She is in great pain and discomfort physically as well as emotionally. There is another factor at play here and in many of these cases. She does not want to be on this kind of medication. People read about the side effects on the Internet and get very alarmed. It is not that they are philosophically against meds. They just don't want to suffer the consequences of them.

I keep a constant fever of 98-99°F. I also have pain in the ankles."

OK, what else?

"I don't eat much anymore. I used to get very high fevers and sweat but not so much anymore. When I get really sick I don't feel like leaving my home, I feel very weak. I am actually afraid to leave the house. I feel safe inside. Six years ago, I was diagnosed with a mild hyperthyroid. The doctor didn't prescribe anything and just recommended rest because I was very stressed. Three years ago, I thought it was back as I was experiencing the same symptoms. I also feel like I cannot run fast and I am losing my memory. I used to get cold (not colds) often when I was a child. I remember now I had a kidney infection when I was eight years old."

Here is the physical process of the attacks she suffers from. She gets freezing cold, and then she starts to shake. After a while the shaking stops and she starts to sweat. Once she sweats the coldness goes away. The shaking is actually an automatic bodily response to create heat within itself. It is the equivalent of rubbing your arms when you feel cold.

(long pause)

Please continue. Could you tell me what is going through your mind at this moment?

"Since the lupus, I have had some uncomfortable dreams. Not scary but feeling like things go wrong. I have a recurring dream. I am not afraid of technology but this dream keeps coming back. Would you like me to tell you about it?

She stopped speaking and seemed to be thinking of something. It is important to respect these moments to allow space for the person to freely go where her instinct tells her. Most of the time though people are just trying to make sure they make sense. Of course, that's not what I am looking for, as it is the brain talking rather than the feelings.
Here she chose to go with her dreams.

Certainly...

"In this dream I live in a tall building. We live on the 3rd floor and the elevator keeps going even past the 12th floor, which is supposed to be the top floor. It is very scary. It is like not knowing what is going on. I keep thinking what is going to happen to me? Maybe it is going to take me up to the sky. It cannot be, it does not exist. There are little windows and I look out because I want to know exactly where I am going."

Pierre: Tell me about your childhood, please.

"It was like living two lives: happy and sad. I had a lot of problems but there was a problem with my father who has a big psychological problem. I suffered from a lot of verbal abuse in the house. I was torn between my mother and my father. My father and I don't need to talk to understand each other. Outside the house everything was great but the stress inside the house was very intense and this is why I left. I really thought my mother was my enemy. I thought my mother might want to kill me, so I left everything behind and left. I had to leave the country because he could have found me anywhere. I get depressed thinking about it. How could I face this mess? I will never feel whole again. Before I left I was diagnosed with hyperthyroid. Every day I spent there was impossible."

At the time, I did not investigate the information in the dream thoroughly enough. Today, it would be totally different. So the next question is very disjointed from the whole.

I understand. Do you have any food cravings?

"I use a lot of salt on everything."

It seems confusing. The father was the abuser but she thought the mother was the enemy. She has a great connection with her father so how could he be the bad guy? What is at play here is that she has resonance with her father.

REMEDY:

Natrum muriaticum

FOLLOW-UP:

Pierre: How are you?

"I have a little more energy than before. The pain in the joints is almost not there and I don't have as many problems when I wake up as I used to. I have had less pain in the joints of the hands. The last few days however have not been as good. I am starting to feel pain in the hands and a little more pain from the skin rash. I had a low grade fever again yesterday. I am afraid now that perhaps it is coming back. I still don't have the chills and I am not shivering but I am concerned as I feel it may be coming back. I have to help my fingers come back from an extended position from time to time but over all it is a better."

Pierre: How about your dream?

"My dreams are much better than the ones I used to have. I have depressing dreams but now they are coming back to the way they were before all this. I feel like the remedy did good but it did not win the war."

REMEDY:

Repeat the remedy

FOLLOW-UP 2 THROUGH 6: (9 months)

"I finished the remedy and altogether I feel better. Mentally I am very comfortable. I

There is nothing stronger than resonance. It is like an electric lock. It looks like one could just be able to pry it open easily but in fact, it is stronger than anything else.

Considering my understanding of the case at the time I asked about the food craving for a confirmation of my choice of remedy. The salt craving indeed confirmed it. The remedy was selected with an analysis like this:
1. I need a remedy with features of icy coldness almost to the point of delirium, but with intermittent heat;
2. Joint pain;
3. The remedy must have grief regarding the mother (Today I would never assume the feeling since it was not spoken in those terms); and,
4. Craving for salt.

These four points represent a totality, not *the* totality.

The remedy had some resonance but clearly the lupus is still there and "coming back."

stopped taking the steroid medication and I started to experience some slight numbness especially in the 3rd and 4th finger but overall I can do without it. At times, I feel some pain in the wrist and in the palm. I have a hard lump in the right palm and some left elbow pain as if it is dislocated but over all the pain is 80% better. I had a bladder infection a couple of weeks ago, which I used to get frequently, with a milky, slightly yellow discharge. I had to go to the bathroom often soon after drinking. I feel like there is something going on with my kidneys like I used to have when I was 8 years old. When I was a child I had a lot of fevers. In one month I had two tonsil infections. I have no more fevers and no shivering cold but I have this odd feeling in that area. Since I started taking the remedy I am the first to get up whereas I could not get out of bed before and I would force myself to sleep. I feel more secure and comfortable about what I have to do. I am more alert. I can remember phone numbers and other things. My dreams are not scary anymore. For example, I had a dream that I am flying like a bird and I am able to escape some problems and fly away. With the lupus I used to have dark colors in my dreams and problems I could not solve but now I can solve the problems. I feel strong and I don't feel tired. I used to always ask for days off, now I can work much more. I can also think so much better, too. I feel more like a whole person. I can choose between things much more easily. I know what I want. The kidney pain is gone. The problem with urination has

Even by today's standards, we would not change the remedy. Lupus is an extremely serious condition and to expect it to be gone in such a short time would not be reasonable.

improved a lot. I thought all my problems were from my kidney but not anymore. I don't sleep well. I have to sleep on the sofa but when I wake up I feel well. I can sleep only seven hours and I am fine. I was losing my hair before the lupus and that seems to be better now. My fingers feel fine. During the winter I got a slight cold, I did not take medication and it went away on its own. I don't think that would have happened before. I would say my general health is good. I do feel like the inflammation is over and what is left is not going to expand. I am not afraid of it anymore."

REMEDY:

I repeated the remedy a few times during that time

FOLLOW-UP: (1 years later)

Pierre: Tell me what is going on, please.

"I have a lot of pain in all the joints. Any kind of movement becomes an unbearable pain and I feel even worse when I lie down. The whole thing is definitely worse when I rest. I wake up because of the pain. Four or five weeks ago I even thought I had a heart attack. I had a lot of stress. I was working constantly. I started to feel pain around the heart, as if there were air bubbles. One other night while I was working hard I felt a strong pain in the chest area, as if a lump of air was pressing against the ribs. It was as if it were pressing toward the front

The resonance is close enough for her to feel better. For most people this would be a good result especially when you consider two facts:
1. The remedy does not cause side effects, and
2. She is not taking steroids.

with a sensation that I had a hole in the back, which lasted three days. I have had dreams of dead bodies, decomposing bodies since then. I know it is a dream but I should not be seeing things like that."

Have you seen a doctor?

"Yes, I did. He did some tests and he said everything was OK. I did not have a heart attack, my heart is fine."

REMEDY:

Zincum metallicum

FOLLOW-UP: (2 months later)

Pierre: How are you feeling?

"I have been much better. I was great until I got an ear infection. For two weeks I was constantly cold and very sensitive to drafts and I could not warm up".

I think you should have called me.

"This was not the same kind of cold as I used to get with the lupus. I had stiffness in the neck and some burning pain on the tip of the shoulder blade and then something extraordinary happened. I was really well for two days and then my feet started to hurt. I could not walk; I could not even touch the ground. It started on the sole of the feet then moved to the top of feet. It was a *"big pain."* I could not touch anything; I could not take a step. I felt very restless. Only hot baths

At the time I, too, thought it was pretty good but we can do better.

I recommended a different remedy because the characteristics are different from prior visit. Dreaming of dead bodies and having a sensation of a hole in her back is all new. She never talked about anything like that before. In this instance, it is what we call an "inter-current" remedy. Nowadays, I seldom make use of that technique.

Had she come to the office at that point I would most likely have given her a remedy called *Rhus toxicodendron*. This remedy has features of restlessness, not being able to sit for any amount of time with excruciating muscle or fascia pain. Only a hot bath gives slight relief but then restlessness and pain quickly

helped. In the morning all the pain was gone. Unfortunately, two weeks later all the pains came back. I am very confused. I can't sleep all night. I am feeling lazy. I have salt cravings again. My brain does not seem to work. I can't do riddles, whereas normally I am very good. I feel indecisive. My husband is a pain, I am not feeling love toward him or others. I am thinking of unpleasant things from the past, what my father said a long time ago, etc. I am not happy."

REMEDY:

Repeat the first remedy given, *Natrum muriaticum.*

FOLLOW UP:

Pierre: Long time no see. How are you feeling?

"Some pains remain but it is mostly a little stiffness. I have had arguments with my husband. I prefer to be by myself and I've come to realize I had almost no relationship with my mother. The flair-ups have not been so severe. The reason why I am here is because I got pregnant. It's a very high-risk pregnancy with a high possibility for genetic complication and I would like to be as well as possible. I had a dream that a little girl was walking towards the light."

REMEDY:

Repeat *Natrum muriaticum*

returns. In other words, it fits exactly what she was describing. I used this remedy myself once after I was shivering cold in a pool while I was trying to impress a girl. The day after I was in screaming, tearing pain. I couldn't hold myself straight; I was going from one hot shower to my bed and back to the shower. Moving about relieved the mental anguish a little but it did not relieve the physical pain much at all. I couldn't get a remedy since I was on a tiny island. I suffered all the way back home on the plane. The first thing I did once I got home two days later was take *Rhus toxicodendron.* I felt relief almost instantly.

We had a long conversation regarding her dream of a guide coming and bringing comfort and reassurance to her that everything will be fine.
Though there were quite a few odds stacked against her everything turned out perfectly fine.

From here on this is the new and far better way of taking a case and analysis.

FOLLOW-UP: (Three years later)

Pierre: How have you been?

"I have had a lot of stress in the last two weeks. I volunteered to run my friend's wedding. It was a lot of work and stress, everything ended up on my shoulders. I did everything by myself *then* my husband came to the wedding and told me that it was "no work, It's not a big deal." I was the leader and when he came and said that it was so destructive. I had planned every little detail with puzzle accuracy. I felt like "You are trying to destroy this perfect puzzle." This is the last day and you come to destroy it. I can't believe he said that even up to now. The only one who did not like it was my husband. I don't know if he did it out of vengeance or stupidity. I think it is vengeance. I am completely shocked to the point that I cannot cry. I was very pleased with the wedding - everybody was - and at the same time I am very dissatisfied with my personal life. I don't know what to do. I think this relationship is not going anywhere if he turns everything to shit. I am very satisfied with myself. I know I may not have a Ph.D. but how can I do this with somebody who contradicts me all the time?"

Describe the feeling of shock a little more, please.

"At first I felt disbelief and then big, big, big anger. It was a huge disappointment. I am afraid now. Do I share my love with the enemy? Obviously, this was planned. I had to put my anger on the back burner at the time

Here we see the theme of enemy that was at the beginning of the case represented by the mother. The feeling of disbelief and leaving mentioned before are there, too. The symptoms of lupus are the same but the deeper feelings were never elucidated. Now the most central remedy, the most similar (simillinum) will have a far deeper effect than any of the others. I need a remedy that has features of being so shocked it is to the point of not being able to cry and that as a result the feeling is complete destruction.

but I now have a constant feeling that I cannot rely on him. Then I got upset that the person I share my life with is helping to destroy it. If someone is jealous of my success I can't stand it. It hurts me that I have to explain this to him. I can feel all the symptoms of lupus coming back; all my pains are coming back. I want to cry but I can't, I can't get my anger out. I would like to but I can't."

Here we can clearly see that up to now the remedy had been palliative only. It never reached the deepest root. Now this remedy is resonating deep into the VF (Vital Force).

REMEDY:

Hoang nan

Pierre: Tell me about the lupus.

"By the time I received the remedy I had all the symptoms of lupus. I was very weak. I didn't eat. I was confused, chilly and I could not get out of bed because of the pains. We were supposed to go Upstate but I stayed home. One day after taking the remedy I went shopping. I felt immediately that the progress of the lupus had stopped. It was like something had lifted."

Tell me more, please.

"I am not in shock anymore. Definitely I can think like I could not before. I have a lot of anger directed at my father. My sister brought pictures and I saw my father. When I left my country, I was not able to deal with him. It was basically emotional abuse so much so that I could not talk about it. I did not have it in order. Now this part is over. I have everything

She has a lot of anger toward her father. These are the first signs of something deeper happening. Her perception is coming into better focus or into "order."

Now this is a deep acting remedy. She sees things as they really are. Her demeanor is far more upbeat, this is a deeply changing individual. This is the first time we are moving away from the physi-

in order. I was a victim of wrongdoing. I don't feel hopeless anymore. I was afraid of going back to my country but not anymore. He's too old to take him on physically but I could confront him now."

I think we are looking at something that is far deeper than before, don't you think?

"When I saw the picture, I got angry at the way my mother looked and I am sure she looks like that because she is with my father. She does not deserve such a life. I have some anger but the feeling of it is not bad, it is certainly better than being afraid. I feel totally better; there is a big difference from before. Even the nodules in my hands are much better. They are gone in the left hand and the right hand is better. I am somebody. I would say this is an active state. I'm thinking a lot about business, I feel I can do something on my own."

What about your husband?

"I told him either we work it out or we split." He said, "OK, I will send you decent child support" so I said, "You don't understand, I go and I send you child support." So he started thinking and now he realizes that it is better not to walk away. I could never have said such a thing before. I am able to say things right, which never happened before. This is becoming a very important point in my life. I could not do business and take care of things because things were not in order and behind

cals and freely exploring the emotional level. That said, the nodules on the fingers were very hard and I too never thought they could go away, let alone so quickly.

I asked about her husband at the end, as I was surprised she did not mention him.

Viva la freedom. Lupus libre! Resonance sets you free.

The remedy was repeated once in six months.

Over the last five years, few symptoms ever flared up and it is clear that the deeper remedy restored her health on a totally different level. All the symptoms of lupus have now clearly disappeared: the fever, the coldness and, as unbelievable as it is, the nodules that had formed in her hands have also disappeared. Her emotional state is clearer and who doesn't need that?

me. I feel younger as if I were 23. I can't believe how old I am."

REMEDY:

Continue

FOLLOW-UP:

Pierre: How are you?

"I am doing very well. Life is good, I am free to pursue anything I like."

REMEDY:

Continue

PHONE:

"I continue to feel very well. There is no lupus."

ERIKA

(Mid 30's)

MC: LUPUS ERYTHEMATOSUS

- Forgetful
- Herpes on the middle finger
- Gastro-esophageal reflux disease (GERD)

Pierre: Tell me about the lupus, please.

"At this point I don't know I am 35 years old, I feel so old. I can't believe I have lupus. There is nothing like that in my ethnic background. I don't think we get it."

I am not sure about ethnic background... but tell me more about the lupus.

"It is ruining my life, my marriage and my daughter. I have very little patience with everyone and I fight with my husband. I want to work out but I can't because it hurts. My left hip and knees hurt. It is absolutely awful and it affects my whole family. I'm always tired and my husband yells because I can't satisfy him. He thinks I am making excuses."

Please continue.

"I wake up in the middle of the night with excruciating pains. I have so much pain in my elbow I can't even extend my arm. When I walk I have pain in the knees and hips yet when I wake up in the morning I don't have any pain. Why is that?"

DISCUSSION

She was diagnosed with Lupus 4 years ago. At first the doctors thought it might be scleroderma because of the severity of her GERD symptoms and other gastro intestinal problems.

As we see throughout the book, we think the person with the problem knows best about her condition. The sufferer might have some technical misconceptions as is the case when she says "I don't think we get it in my ethnic background" but deep down in the individual constitution there is no doubt that only the person experiencing the ailment is the one who can describe it.

It is unusual for people to start describing the way the condition is affecting them. I ask her to tell me more about the lupus and she tells me "it is ruining my life." Most of the time people ease into it by talking about the physical symptoms rather than the emotional state. Either way it is fine by me because the road map of case taking is very clear, only the destina-

I will explain later, please continue I don't want to lose the flow of this.

"At around 3 or 4 a.m. I wake up with this constant, severe pain that feels as if it is sitting in the elbow, as though something is in there. Something wants to torture me. It is a torture. The whole lupus feels like I am being punished. I am not worthy of having a normal life. This thing is tightening in my elbow as if it were torture. It takes a grip of the elbow and it won't let go. I think it comes on suddenly but I don't know how because it happens while I am sleeping and then it wakes me up."

Tell me more about how all this is affecting you, please.

"All the things I like to do I can't do. It is ruining my life. I lose my patience easily. My husband thinks the lupus is an excuse. It is very hard to live like that, I mean, if there is a little wind on the elbow I hurt, that's how sensitive it is at this point. The coldness of it makes it worse. It is as if my elbow is made of metal."

(She pauses and thinks.)

"I was born breached, my left side has always been much weaker than the right. My muscles just don't support the joint and I feel very unstable. I think that's how I am in my head, too. It's like the left side is worse than the right. When I walk, my left side is much more painful than the right. I also have a pain that radiates down the leg as if someone were

tion is not known until the end of the consultation.

Very often people ask me, "Why is this happening?" I never answer these questions. There are two practical reasons for that. It is best to continue with the story rather than give an answer that in the end has little or no relevance. Secondly, it is up to a doctor to respond to these inquiries.

Some people might think that the on again/off again nature of the symptoms as they are stated in the previous answer might be a psychosomatic complaint. It could not be further from the truth. Rather this on/off characteristic is part of the experience of the disorder.

I never know where the case takes me. It is all part of the story, which as a homeopath I always find interesting. Let's see if "being born breached" leads anywhere and if somehow it relates...

pushing a nail inside my left hip. It is a very sharp pain."

Tell me about feeling unstable, please.

"I have always been. I was born with a weaker left side. I never did any sport because of that. When I swim, I always have to adjust to stay in the lane. If it weren't for the lane buoy I would swim in a circle. I also think that's how I am. Within a day I go up and down. I can't live like this. It is because of that unstable feeling that I feel responsible for being happy and unhappy with my family. I also try to do more for others, I obsess about the house being clean."

You are doing a great job. Please continue.

"I have one strong side and one weak side. With me, it has always been uneven. I am hot or cold, for example. I am nice and then I yell. I cover just my feet and then I cover my whole self. My feet get cold and then hot. I cover myself entirely then I am too warm."

Let's go back to how this is affecting you, please.

"I can't do things I love to do. I feel like I am crippled. I am trying to avoid how it will be. It makes me angry."

Describe the feeling, please.

"I get pissed or I take a nap. I am no good anymore. I can't fix it. I feel guilty. I would like

The feeling of "being unstable" relates to a larger totality comprising the lupus with the emotional state that accompanies it. It is a characteristic symptom once the feeling of being unstable is recognized as being on the physical or emotional level.

Do notice that the suggestion "Tell me about being unstable" is not a leading question. It is very important that it be so to give the most freedom for answering according to the disorder in the constitution. No one can assume to know what should come next.

When she says, "I am cold or hot. I have one strong side and one weak one," it reminds me of the on and off symptoms she described earlier in the case.

Here we have the ruined feeling again, so it means a lot.

to be a good mother but the lupus has really ruined my life. When my husband says it's just an excuse, I feel even more guilty. I feel guilty that I have ruined things for my daughter and for him. It gets darker and darker; it is like being in a well. It gets deeper and deeper. It is slow like Chinese torture. I am worn out and terribly worried about it. I can't keep fighting it. I hurt all over; even my nails and my hair hurt. I feel so helpless."

Valerie had the same feeling of "being ruined." In Valerie's case, it took a long time to "extract the root" whereas in this case it was mentioned right at the beginning (see case). Though the root feeling is similar, there is still a drastic difference in the way the condition is perceived. Here she is helpless; in Valerie's case she feels it is hopeless.

Can you tell me more? Please continue.

"I am very agitated and restless. My thoughts are racing non-stop. What am I going to do? Outside I look calm but inside I am tired. Inside I am constantly shivering, as if I had too much coffee and there is constant trembling. I am never steady. I would like to be calm. It is like my heartbeat, it is up, up, up, up and then it goes down but never to a baseline. I feel like it is running on empty. I look for distracters to this whole thing. I try to hold two jobs. I have my kid, three dogs and a rabbit. I feel like I am drowning, falling in a well as I mentioned."

This is very serious. She is telling more now about how systemic the pain really is. There is pain even in her nails and hair.

Tell me about your dreams, please.

"I am sleeping. I am gasping for air. I can't move. I want to fight but I can't. I am doing it with all my might, so much effort but I can't. I am fighting for my life but I can't get out. This is weird, the feeling that I have of having lupus is the same."

At this point I thought I knew the remedy she needed so I looked for more information in a different direction to cross my "T's" and dot my "I's." I asked her about her dreams and, as you can see, the dreams give the same feeling as in life so we have come full circle. If my analysis is correct the remedy should start lifting the disorder very quickly.

Tell me about the feeling of being ruined, please.

"I am angry about it. There is so much trembling and then it goes, I don't stop it. It goes on its own."

REMEDY:

Cimicifuga racemosa

FOLLOW-UP: (one month)

Pierre: Can you tell me how you are?

"There is a huge difference, really huge. Everything became alive. I was so hopeless. I see the difference. I felt wonderful within 3 or 4 days and after that I felt a little pain come back. Then after two weeks I felt better again."

That's *good*. What else has happened?

"My hip and elbow pains are gone. I wake up at 3:22 AM every morning until 5 AM. My thoughts are racing but I don't have any pain now. I had difficulty walking up and getting out of bed before I came to see you and now I go to the gym. I don't feel as cold on the outside and hot on the inside as I used to either. Also, the sensation of having a sharp nail in the hip is totally gone. I feel my left side is stronger. I am so amazed, I don't even think about my left side now."

Tell me more about what is better and not better.

"My heartbeat is calmer, the palpitations don't happen as often. I don't feel as down, I don't

The remedy seems clear.

I love quick action; at the same time I don't expect it. Isn't the reversal of so much disorder really mind opening to the possibilities and to what it is that ails us?

Because the left side had been such a long standing complaint we know for sure the remedy is acting very deeply.

feel like I am getting deeper and deeper in the well. My nails and hair pain is totally gone. The shivering has also much improved. My marriage problems are better at this moment. I had filed for divorce but we made up so perhaps there is some hope. I am feeling responsible for him. I wake up at 3:22 a.m. and I think about it. On the other hand, my relationship with my daughter is much better; I don't lose my temper as much. It is really wonderful. I am also not as tired, which really helps when you have a young child."

Anything else?

I don't think so. Oh, the skin on my middle finger is much better, too, but not totally gone."

SUMMARY OF SEVERAL FOLLOW-UPS:

"The racing thoughts are much better. I am still very good overall. The weakness on the left side continues to improve. Shivering and night sweats are pretty much gone. I noticed my memory is much better. The skin on my finger continues to get better. My relationship with my daughter continues to improve. I don't know what is going to happen with my husband at this moment. I don't wake up as much at night as I used to so I guess I am not as concerned about it."

What is deeply satisfying in doing this work is that I see a lot of people who can't be helped with medicine and they return to a vibrant state of health. It speaks as to the beauty of homeopathy. In this case, the remedy matched her to a T and very good results were achieved. Some might ask do you have a remedy for everyone or everything? Of course we can't do everything. This is not miraculous work, but it is wise to give it a fair try.

Better down to the last possible details.
The follow-ups are absolutely crucial for case management. Many people think that as they are better physically there is no need to continue. This is not true. Health is not static. It really ebbs and flows all the time much like the day one is diagnosed is not the day one became sick. It is a process that starts many years prior. Bringing health back is a process of reversal. I see it as rolling a train back. First there needs to be a slow down and then a stop and then the roll back to the start. Discontinuing homeopathy at the time of full stop is not optimal.
I continued the same remedy in different potencies according to what was going on.
The marriage did not survive. My view on that is that the decision was taken from a healthy point of view rather than a "ruined" point of view.

LAHAR
(Early 30's)

DISCUSSION

MC: MASTITIS

• Deep anger

Pierre: You told me on the phone you are in great pain, please tell me about it.

"I feel sick and I can't get out of it; it feels as if my body is shutting down. I have a cracked nipple and at times it is bloody. I am breastfeeding. My doctor said it is mastitis. It started in the right breast, then the left breast started to act up with enormous pain. It is extremely sensitive. When the right duct was blocked I was screaming as if I were delivering. Now the left breast hurts and it is bleeding. It is an enormous pain and it's extremely sensitive. I am so tired of the pain I can't bear it anymore. I am feeling sick and stressed; it's not like me at all. I had mastitis before but I could do everything I needed to do. This time I can't."

Could you tell me more about the sensitivity?

"This time the sensitivity disturbs me and it burns. I don't like to suffer. At this moment it is the only thing I think about. I can't control the suffering. It is a rather vicious pain. It is so intense, like a strong stabbing pain. I can't concentrate on anything. I feel like I am losing my head to it. I go in a room and I forget what I came in for."

I present this case because the intensity of the physical pain matches the intensity of the emotional and mental level. This is common but we never quite see it that way. It is generally "lost in translation" as I call it. Lost in translation means that the inter-intensity as well as the inter-connectivity of the PEM is not acknowledged within the connected whole. At best, in the alternative world there is a disconnected whole where one can make lifestyle changes, often with great efforts to achieve limited results. With homeopathy it is not the case. We do not ask people to make changes. We approach this matter as the changes should happen from the inside out. The inside is where the strength really is. In that sense, a frail looking body with a strong life force on all levels is better than a big body with a frail Vital Force.

The spontaneous choice of words is always very interesting because they are the only way to transport us into the interior. Here she

186

Please, tell me more about the suffering.

"I have a phobia of mice and rats. After my daughter's birth, I had anxieties that someone was going to take her. I get out of the shower just to check on her. I found mouse droppings in my house, in my basement, and I completely freaked out then I saw a dead mouse in the yard. Yesterday I was lying down in bed and I thought somebody was cutting my daughter's arm. I know it sounds extreme, but that's what is going on. I feel very protective of her. I could have extreme anger if anybody did anything to her; I could kill an elephant. I have always been very violent. I like to hurt and get hurt. I fought against much stronger boys than I in school. I used to be violent, and I used to have violent thoughts upon myself. This is the only way I could have intercourse. I was abused and terrified of sexual thought, then it turned and I was very promiscuous. I can't stand surprise; it's like a mouse that arrives at any time. Rats, really disgust me. Even in a coloring book they disgust me. I feel like they are going to dirty me. I feel like they are going to climb on me, and touch me, and bite me. I saw one a long time ago and I cried for four hours. I am absolutely terrified."

Please tell me about being horrified.

"It is horrible suffering. I can take so much but at that moment it feels like a huge creature eating people with limbs flying. I know I am going to suffer but I can only take so much."

uses the word "vicious" and "strong stabbing pain." These words are very telling of the nature of the disorder. As the case goes on, we'll see how important what "lost in translation" really is. "Lost in translation" makes me think of fishermen who used to use lobster for bait until they realized how good it really is and how much people liked it once introduced to it. It is all around us but we just don't notice it.

As we see over and over in these cases, seemingly disconnected features are threaded into the condition with no apparent logic and yet it leads to the root that brought all of it up in the first place. Here she is talking about her extreme fear of rats and the potential rage in

Talk to me about fighting.

"It removes all the hate I have in me. When I'm fighting, I control the situation. As soon as the anger takes over I am invincible. I just see red with anger to the tips of my fingers. All that is needed is a trigger. I very rarely have repentance. Whatever has been done should not have been done. The pain in the breast I can't control, the pain from a fight I can. When I suffer I am not mean; I am not violent with the people I love."

Could you describe these feelings a little more, please.

"When I fight I control the situation, I have no respect for men, and it is extremely intense. At times, I feel like some people put me in a little girl state. When my parents somewhat acknowledged the problem of me being abused, I felt on the side. I came home and went to my room. I felt rejected. I felt that I must be a real shit for them not to pay attention to it. I did not feel part of the family. I couldn't spit at his face or kill him."

REMEDY:

Lyssinum

FOLLOW-UP:

Pierre: How are you feeling?

her. The question was about "suffering." An open question and letting her describe the web of her suffering takes us straight down the Golden Thread all the way to the root of her ill.

What is really great about this case is that the intensity is beautifully well reflected on all levels: Physical, emotional and mental.

189 CASES FROM MY PRACTICE

"I have been feeling very calm, I am not so quick to anger. The violent thoughts are also better. The anger that I had to hit someone is also better. I am capable of concentrating. My breasts started to feel fine immediately after I took the remedy and I have been able to breastfeed without any problems. I had blocked ducts for a very short time once. Rats or mice don't seem to cause as many anxieties as before. I actually saw a mouse in a field close to my house, but I did not have the feeling that it was going to jump on me. That anxiety became slightly more intense after I took the remedy. Now it is much better."

REMEDY:

Continue

SEVERAL FOLLOW-UPS:

"Rats used to be repulsive to me whereas they are okay now. Sex has been good, absolutely no problem whatsoever, whereas for years I was in therapy and it didn't do anything. I have not had any thoughts of anyone taking my daughter and I have not had any violent thoughts. At some point I had a lot of vaginal discharge, which took two weeks to improve on its own. I am feeling very well. I used to have really strange thoughts during intercourse, now I no longer have them."

There is nothing quicker to restore health than the right remedy acting in similarity upon the Vital Force.

KESHIA

(Late 50's)

MC: MIGRAINES

- Headaches
- Frequent colds
- Allergies
- Insomnia
- Prescription drug addiction

Pierre: We spoke about migraines on the phone, is that right?

"Yes, but the temptation to start pain killer medication again is very strong, if I could get these meds I would, on the other hand, my granddaughter is the light of my life and she said I would not be able to see her by myself if I did so. That is the only reason why I don't take them. My whole family knows I am addicted to this stuff. It is an addiction; that is why they won't let me see her if I take them."

I see...

"I haven't gone out of my house for the last two months. I am really afraid of going back to medication. I need help and I don't know what to do. I was always energetic and a good mother, it's only in the last couple of years that I have been sleeping all the time. I don't want to go the psychiatrist because they give medications but then by the same token my husband does not like my therapist. I am supposed to go away on a trip at the end

DISCUSSION

I present this case to show the necessity of keeping up with the follow-ups. It may sound obvious but some people don't do it. It is a mindset from the medical establishment, one gives a remedy and that should be that. I believe this lady could be a lot better but without follow-ups it is impossible. What happens sometimes is that people don't quite understand what we are doing. "How could this little remedy do so much? For so long the doctors have tried everything." Indeed, it is mind boggling for some people. The remedy comes in a granule half the size of a Tic Tac. If it is liquid, it only takes a few drops under the tongue. This is what chapter two of this book explains. My answer to this is "Size doesn't have anything to do with it. Accuracy has everything to do with it."

The addictive nature of these medications to wreck a family is evident here.

of May, but I think what if the headaches or migraines come on, what am I going to do?"

Tell me about your migraines, please.

"They usually start while I am sleeping around 3 or 4 AM. By 6 AM I feel sick to my stomach and I have to go the bathroom. Once the migraine starts, it last approximately 14 hours. I must tell you that I never feel good overall these days and I don't know why. Why is this happening to me? I just wish I could feel better about myself. I want to be normal again. I have lost so much weight. I feel 20 years older than I really am. I always felt like a good mother; when my son had some special needs I became PTA president so that he would get a proper education. For someone who always tries to do the right thing and help others, I am feeling mentally weak. I am hurting my family but there are various different kinds of addictions in my family and I feel very embarrassed. I'll tell you what. I always wanted to be a nurse but my girlfriends told me so many things about it that I withdrew my application. I was over 50 when I went back to school for it. The professor made one remark and I dropped out. What I do now is not satisfying me. I don't know what else I can say to explain what I have done, or what I have been through, I need help."

The "Why me?" feeling although not very strong here is a very common one. It is human nature to ask the question, "Why me?" when something is wrong. Often the answer is "I have been a good person" or "I am being punished." People often take themselves through either one of these two emotions during the consultation but "Why?" generally leads to rationalization which is not very useful for our purpose. What I look for is more of a spontaneous, instinctual feeling.

In many ways there is a strong theme of nurturing here but I need to figure out the feeling behind it.

Well, let's start with the feeling of needing help.

"I have always been the one to be there for others. When I was nineteen my father died, and I took over his stuff because my mother was out of it, she couldn't deal with anything. The only time I am happy is when I am watching my granddaughter. Most of the time I want to cry and cry and cry a lot. Everything bothers me, I am letting everybody down, it was always the opposite. I just don't understand what is going on with me."

Describe the feeling of letting everyone down.

"I am not supposed to do that. I am supposed to make people happy. I have been like this since I was a child, it was expected of me. I was always the one who came through. By eight years of age, I ironed, washed, cooked, and I took care of my brother. I did things without being asked. I wanted to please. I would have done anything to make everybody happy. If I didn't please them, I thought I was doing something wrong and I felt rejected."

Her story of being a young child with some responsibilities towards others in the family is surprisingly quite common, even in the U.S.

Tell me more about your migraines.

"I have had migraines since the headaches started. It's always on the left side, and it is better if I lie down. Coffee or Coca-Cola makes it a little bit better. I never want to eat with the migraines; I only want to vomit while I have them."

I wanted to know a lot more about the need to please and nurture people. I needed to see how that related to the migraines but she was very reluctant to talk so I gave a remedy the old-fashioned way by picking a few symptoms and cross-referencing them. This is a very valid way of analyzing this case. It simply is not the latest way of doing things. It helped.

REMEDY:

Cocculus (See comments)

FOLLOW-UPS:

Pierre: How are you feeling?

"The headaches are not as bad. It seems as if the remedy has kept them under control. I have had no sick headaches as I call them and no migraines. I have been sleeping much better and I fall asleep rather well, now. The temptation of taking medication is still there, although not having the headaches did lessen the temptation. I did not notice any change emotionally, but I must say that in many ways I feel generally much better."

Feeling better physically is great. Feeling better emotionally is wonderful and feeling mentally better is fantastic. If the follow-ups are kept up, wholesome beautiful health springs forth. It is a deep and secured feeling not just a little alleviation. If a little alleviation feels that great, imagine how much more can be achieved. In this case we have the added problem of prescription drug addiction. I can't imagine the remedy restoring health for any amount of time longer than a few months under these circumstances. But *c'est la vie*. You didn't think a Frenchman writing a book in English would not say that once, did you?

TOM

(Late 20's)

MC: MIGRAINES

- Chronic sinusitis for 15 years
- Low energy, needs to take naps
- Lower back and knees weakness
- Sensation of blocked hearing

Pierre: I understand you have chronic sinusitis.

"Yes I do. The pressure at the root of my nose is very bad in the morning when I wake up. I sneeze several times in the morning and I have to blow my nose a bunch of times before stringy mucus comes out. I feel better after sneezing but I constantly hear a whistle sound in the nose when I breathe. The pain gets really bad with cold weather and it is definitely better in warm weather. Cold weather also gives me a blinding headache. If I apply some pressure on the nose it gets a little bit better for a short time."

You also mentioned migraines, please tell me about them.

"Yes, I think they are related to eating meat and or drinking milk after which I get a massive visual disturbance and dizziness. I get very sensitive to light and sound and then I vomit. The pain always affects one side the left or the right side but never both at the same time."

DISCUSSION

Tom was diagnosed with migraines 8 yrs prior to seeing me.

I present this case to show that self-prescribing with homeopathic remedies for a chronic condition is not very effective. He has taken several homeopathic remedies on his own such as Kali bichromatum and Hydrastis. One can find a lot of information about remedies online but it is close to impossible to be accurate. If you have a cold or a minor issue, then by all means take a crack at it, but for anything else, please see a professional classical homeopath. I do not intend to be patronizing but a good homeopath is able to resolve problems more efficiently.

I asked a lot of questions regarding the sinusitis but beyond what we have here not much more information was coming forward hence no conclusive remedy could be found.

It is possible to arrive at the correct remedy through any ailments because ultimately the root of the disorder is the same. One person with several ailments equals one root. It is Tom who walks in the consultation room not sinusitis holding hands with migraine accompanied by lower back pain. In a situ-

Is there a pattern to it? Does it start on the right and then goes to the left or any other way? Alternating perhaps?

"I looked for that for so long but it is totally haphazard. I tried so many times to see if there is a pattern but I have not seen one."

OK, let's continue with the migraines. Please tell me more about them.

"I just want to sleep and sip some water while I have them. After sleeping a whole night there is a residual pain when I shake my head or when I bend forward. About two years ago, I started to wake up with a headache and acid reflux. That's headache though, they don't have anything to do with the migraines."

I understand, please tell me about the migraines.

"As far as the migraines are concerned the pain is generally around the eyes. It feels very deep, it comes and goes for about 10-second intervals. It seems like it lets up and then it comes back. The migraines start as soon as I wake up. Lights or brightness get magnified. My vision is not affected, it just feels like my eyes are being subjected to a type of brightness that is like an interrogation lamp. It makes me feel like I am suffocating. The onset is very sudden. It really gets me in a strong and powerful way."

ation like this it is easier to get to the root by way of his migraines because migraines are so painful the sufferer has more to gain by getting rid of them than by getting rid of a low grade sinusitis.

By asking a question about patterns I am trying to see if there is anything Strange, Rare and Peculiar (SRP). I can quickly discern that and it would afford me a shortcut to the remedy. It is a try but it rarely works. It is a little bit like the husband driving and promising his wife he has a shortcut. It is rarely so.

He is weaving his answers with other ailments. That's very good though it can get confusing. The golden thread, as I often call it in this book, takes us to all the physical issues through the emotional level and on to the mental plane. People often have a difficult time transitioning into feelings. I ask, "What is the feeling?" How do the migraines feel not only physically but also emotionally to him. "How do they affect you?" I mentioned at the beginning of this case that one can look at the remedies online in what we call *Materia Medicas*. MM's are encyclo-

Tell me more about "it gets you in a strong and powerful way".

"When it happens I have to sit down. The nausea sets in and I am not able to do anything. I can't talk to anyone. It feels better if I lay down on my back. Sound gets magnified just like light does. Something is being held in a state of pain." **(He is making a gesture of making a fist opening and closing.)**

Please tell me more about that state of pain.

"In 1997 I had some financial stress. I felt guilty about not being able to make ends meet by myself. I felt I let my parents down because I studied theater. I was anxious and I had fear about the future."

OK, I would like you to tell me more, please.

"I prefer to do one task detailed and organized rather than multi-task which I am not really able to do. I need the breathing room. When I multi-task, I get anxious and nervous as if I were drinking coffee."

How do the migraines affect you, please.

"I need to be left alone. I become irritable, I cannot think as fluently and I feel as if my stomach is held in. I feel really bad in crowded spaces. I get a little edgy and I have a draining feeling in the lower back and in the knees. In 1991, I suffered a massive accident that left me with little feeling in the hand. I can't use

pedias, some as large as 12 volumes, where symptoms of all kinds are noted and described. There can literally be hundreds of symptoms for one remedy and we have thousands of remedies. It is like searching for a needle in a haystack. The way I go about finding a remedy is very different than just looking up physical symptoms and cross referencing remedies a couple of remedies. My process involves discerning the precise pattern encompassing the totality of the encroachment on the PEM levels. As I mentioned before, one needs a professional. To give you an example I don't nor can I take my own case.

He is talking to me about multi-tasking in the kitchen. You might ask yourself "How is this relevant?" You're right. It may not lead anywhere for the purpose of finding a remedy. This makes me think about something I hear every day. A lot of people are concerned about what they say. People say "I am not sure if this right," or "Am I telling you what you need to hear?" Don't be concerned about it. If the answer doesn't lead anywhere it will reveal itself as such. In this case, after a couple of questions, I chose to take a couple of steps back and ask: "How do the migraines affect you?"

my hand as well as the other. I get very nervous about it. It is as if I had too much coffee."

As if too much coffee?

"I like to have intensity and passion of things. The down side of this intensity is that I can take only a little of it at one time. I like to plan things, when is the car going to pick me up, for example? When I cook, I need to have all the ingredients lined up. If not, I feel like I'm losing control. With the migraine I have an empty feeling in my stomach around my belly button and an open feeling when it is not tightening or held in."

Tell me a little more about the feeling of being "held in."

"I never want to be talked to. The feeling is the opposite of free, open space, fluidity, accessible, communicate, letting go, not having the mind involved, openness. The feeling of being held in feels like closing in, holding pressure. My father was very domineering. I had the sense that I was wrong and screamed at all the time. I always have this fear of being dominated and I have a fear of outbursts. I am holding tension in my head, eyes and stomach. I feel a tightening. I have a fear of being in that situation again. Sometimes I have a distinct feeling that my hair is more alive and that I am more present and aware of it."

When he says, "held in" a second time he used the same hand gesture of closing and opening his fist as he did the first time. In my work of distilling everything down to what ties everything together, movements or gestures of the hands while describing feelings becomes very interesting and important. When people start putting the pain in motion the whole condition becomes dynamic. Since it is the Vital Force we are interested in, it makes sense that we wait for it to express itself before we do anything else. As we have seen dynamis (VF) needs to be met by a dynamic substance, a homeopathic remedy. It is the resonance of the remedy upon the VF that returns the VF to a state of health.

The open and tightening feeling he is talking about clearly matches the hand gesture.

He has "fears of outbursts." Outbursts here mean opening as in the opposite of "held in," therefore it is the same feeling. We are not losing anything in the translation between physical and emotional.

Now the feeling of tightening is combining with a feeling in childhood. The process

Please tell me more about this "opening and closing." (I make the same gesture he made.)

"When I do feel open I almost don't have feeling in my body. It just feels good, as if the eyes have opened up like a flower. It is really fluid."

Tell me more about being fluid.

"It is like a strong active meditative state. There is one single coordinated flow. A walk in the park becomes an incredible thing. I am immediately able to listen to music. It is really great but it doesn't happen often."

REMEDY: (1 month)

Opuntia vulgaris

FOLLOW UP:

Pierre: How are you, how are you feeling?

"The first week after I took the remedy I felt a little tingling on the left side of my neck and head. I should point out that I used to have something similar years ago. I got some hot flashes on the side of my head too but it all felt satisfying."

Are you congested in the morning?

"The day after I took the remedy I got up with a lot of nasal congestion and I felt the mucus drain in my throat. That same day I got a migraine but could go on with the day and

of spiraling down to the root is happening very neatly. Let me point out again that this is not psychotherapy and that not all cases go back to childhood.

According to his descriptions of the migraine, how it affects him, what it is like and the sensation of what it feels like, I was confident I knew the remedy he needed not only for his migraines but all the other complaints.

even attended a conference, that's really a first."

OK, and after that?

"After two weeks I felt some tiredness again in the lower back, knees and back which to a large degree felt the same as before. I also felt depressed as if the body was going through a shift so I thought things were getting better but now it seems as if all my complaints are still there only to a much lesser degree. I have not had any major attack of sinusitis. I only had one migraine since I took the remedy whereas they used to be several times a week. Work has become a lot easier because of the feeling of being held in comes but moves out quickly and does not affect my focus. I can keep my mind on a problem even with it."

REMEDY:

Continue

SEVERAL FOLLOW UPS LATER:
(8 months)

"Although the migraines got better they did not completely disappear. The held-in sensation I spoke about when I first came to see you is still there. Everything better, everything feels to a lesser degree but everything is still there."

REMEDY:

Cactus grandiflorus

All complaints are better. There is no need to change the remedy. I stayed with the same remedy and the same potency.

He was at a point when he reported one migraine every 3 to 4 weeks. Compared to before, this is a major improvement. The "held in" sensation did not improve any further so I needed to rethink the remedy. I settled on a remedy of the same botanical family with the same opening and closing feature but slightly different qualities. This is like in Bruce's case of IgA nephropathy (see case). A little change and...

That was it! Truth be told, looking back the clues to find the best remedy were right in the first intake. The results are great now but I don't want anyone to think that conditions improved so perfectly as I describe in this

FOLLOW UP: (a few months later)

"Overall there has been a huge improvement. There have been huge improvements in the way I handle tasks, relationships and social interaction. Even my teeth feeling long is better. I never mentioned that because I didn't think anything could be done about it. Everything is better. Now I don't even think I need control. I was thinking about these migraine attacks I used to get and how I had no ability to match their strength. It was so extreme, I felt so helplessness. I am glad it has all gone away."

SEVERAL FOLLOW UPS (over a few years)

"I remain migraine free. They have not been a problem whatsoever. I came back recently because I had flashbacks of the accident but that has totally gone. I feel freed from my father's issues."

book every time. Here we waited about 8 months before I changed the remedy. I tried different potencies taken in various different ways. One does not jump from one remedy to the next quickly, especially with that much improvement. It is a deeply thought out process. I guess what I am trying to say is: "Don't be impatient."

This man now comes about once a year. He remains migraine- and sinusitis free.

NANETTE

(Early 30's)

MC: ARTHRITIS IN THE NECK

(And most other joints)

- Gastro enteritis
  - Vertigo

Pierre: What brings you here?

"My state of health has not been very good for some time now. I have tingling in the hands that comes and goes especially in the evening and in the morning. I also have some pain up in the arm and arthritis in the neck. The skin of my hands is very dry; in fact, I feel like my whole body is dry. I caught a cold recently and I lost my voice. I am also battling a gastro-enteritis since my vacation in Spain and I am not able to eat. My stomach gets very hard. I feel my body is in full change and that's not for the better. "

Fine, is there a precise time when all of this started?

"The arthritis began after something happened professionally. I was supposed to get a promotion and I did not get it. I had to fight for something that should have happened automatically. When there is something wrong with me it goes to my skin. My body has always been sensitive but now it is much worse. I felt manipulated."

DISCUSSION

When Nanette first came to see me she could hardly turn her head. She had to turn her whole body to look at me instead. At her age, to have arthritis is really tragic.

I present this case for the simple reason that arthritis is not an end in itself. Much can be done as in this case. I don't see any reason for people in their 30's to be crippled by such calamity.

We see in both cases of IBS, that the food supply is very compromised. As a matter of public health, it is very difficult to control the millions of tons of food that are produced. Most people at home wash their food but restaurants don't do it as thoroughly as they should mainly for expediency. Hygiene is the biggest food problem facing us at this moment.

Tell me about fighting for that please.

"There is all this stuff coming at me, my promotion. My body is changing and I don't I like it. It is changing in a way that mimics my adolescence. I have teeth and gas problems like a baby. It puts me in this fear. It is something I have had all the time. It is something that can't be controlled."

Tell me about the arthritis, please.

"I am getting arthritis, that's what the doctor told me. It feels as if something is crunching in me. When I am in pain I think, 'What is it going to be like when I get older?' After all I am in my early 30's and my mother has something just like that but for her it started in her late 40's. So I think I am worse off than she."

Please tell me what these changes feel like.

"They feel like my body is going to transform and collapse. My body wants to go one way, my head another and I need to stop for a second. I feel like I have to glue myself back together. It is as if I need to put the head and the body back together."

Could you please describe that in a little more detail?

"It feels as if it is the beginning of vertigo. For example, if I walk fast I need to stop. The head goes faster than the body. When I take the train I feel the vibration on the track a lot. Or, when I go to sleep I feel like going into my

"My body... mimics my adolescence...like a baby...my promotion (at work)."
Within a couple of sentences we have babyhood, adolescence, the promotion and the fear she has had all the time. Wow! That's retracing. Many cases in this book show that but this one is the most succinct in its description.

Up to now we could have thought this is psychosomatic, right? Her arthritis started after she didn't get a promotion. Not getting a promotion was a trigger but the pistol was already loaded. Her mother has the same condition so now we might think this is genetic but as I mentioned in Launa's case of post partum depression (see case), genetic is not engraved in stone either. There is hope! A lot of genetic is transferred according to the state of the Vital Force. Once this is remedied properly there is nothing to fear. At the level of the VF arthritis is the same as bulimia. For example, we have generational bulimia now. In other words the mother is bulimic and the state is transferred to the child. Arthritis is the same. Instead of an emotional / mental level disorder as is the case with bulimia with arthritis we have a physical VF disorder. After the proper remedy the state of Vital Heredity can begin to lift as is explained in Chapter

body to incarnate really very deeply. It feels like I am in this half awake state and I hear wailing inside my body. When I had this crisis at work my tongue was swelling."

Tell me about vertigo please.

"In vertigo one does not have a center. It is if one is being twisted. You are not straight. You can't see the world, you are lonely, lost and abandoned. The spine becomes encroached like a witch. The vertebrae make a squeaky noise and lack articulation. It becomes deformed and fritters away. It all falls apart in pieces, it's all coming apart."

REMEDY:

Physostigma

FOLLOW UP: (One month later)

Pierre: How you are. Have you noticed any improvements?

"The tingling in the hands and the dryness is about the same but my stomach is a lot better. I think my body is in full change. I cried for two days after I took the remedy. I realized that having so much control over everything is not quite the best way to live. What kind of living is this? It made me think about my whole body since my birth. My mental disposition is very different. Now my body is connected with my brain. I am cool about things in general, that's what changed mainly. My body is less reactive to things. I am feeling much calmer."

3 and the next generation can experience greater health.

"I don't have a center... it all falls apart." She feels she is literally falling apart. But there is a deeper level than that. What is the sensation of falling apart? The bones are crumbling.

If she describes this in her thirties like she says, "how am I going to be when I get old?" The sweetness of homeopathy to bring her health back is sweet indeed.

"My body is connected to my brain... I am feeling much calmer." This is an example of a deep reaction on two of the three levels we deal with. The arthritis itself is also getting better. During the initial interview she had mentioned very early memories about her body. The remedy is retracing them to erase them.

You are feeling connected now?

"The need to glue myself back is a lot better. The feeling as if I were dizzy is a lot better, my head, too, as well as the body issues. When I move now there is an alignment within. The feeling of falling is very much improved.

This is very important to me because it was the center of the case.

What about the wailing when falling asleep, please?

"The wailing when falling asleep is also a lot better. It seems that I had some unexpressed things in my life."

How about frittering away?

"The feeling of the lack of articulation (her range of motion) in the vertebrae and the feeling of it frittering away is a lot better. Something has also opened up in the hips. Overall, I feel my health is a lot better. The arthritis in the hands, arms and neck is much better. Only the skin needs to get better."

FOLLOW UP: (Six months later)

Pierre: How are you?

"The shift that happened after I first took the remedy is holding. There is space for new stuff. The heaviness I had is totally better. Most of the arthritis is better. There is a little tension in my jaw and a little cracking in the finger.

Retracing or reverse order of complaints as they came through life is very common in homeopathy. We even have a term for it. We call it Hering's Rule of Cure. When it happens it goes like this: The disorder lessens — from top to bottom, from inside out, from more vital to less vital organs, and from mental to emotional to physical.

Nature has perfectly logical order. There is an order to illness; it cannot be any other way. Nothing is haphazard as we can see over and over throughout these cases. One could say that it is an orderly disorder. This is one of the reasons why homeopaths don't interfere with illness but rather re-establish order in the Vital Force.

The skin has progressively gotten better overtime. As it is suggested above, the skin being the most superficial, it is the last organ to get better.

My stomach is feeling a lot better. The skin problems I had all went away. There is some dizziness still from time-to-time, especially if I turn the head to the right. The feeling of frittering away in the bones is gone. I can move my back, I can turn, bend forward and to the side with little problem."

ROGER

(Late 20's)

DISCUSSION

MC: TOTAL NUMBNESS IN THE FINGERS

• Ringing in the ear

I present this case because it goes back 11 years and it includes a follow-up nine years later. It is sweet and short and demonstrates the beauty of homeopathy. The interview was not nearly as developed as it in Valerie or Erika's lupus case (see case). At the time, we did not look at the totality as deeply as we do now. Nonetheless the results were good albeit not as consistent as they are today.

Pierre: How can I help you?

"I have had a total lack of feeling in my fingertips for years. They are numb. I also have some ringing in the right ear; the sound is very high pitched. I also feel like I have water in the ear. I just don't hear silence."

Can you tell me a little bit about you when this started?

"I used to party all the time because I did not like what I was doing. At the time, I felt trapped doing just one thing, whereas I like to do many things. I was very dissatisfied. I did not like the structure and the regimented ways of my old job. I like what I do now, I am an artist."

OBSERVATION: He appears structured, regimented and tense. It is paradoxical to what he is saying hence it is interesting.

What can you tell me about yourself, please?

'I like to use big words that people don't understand. I also like unusual things. My mother was very disorganized, and I moved in with my father because he was more structured. My father would yell at me all the time and I would hide in the house. He was totally structured and regimented. Recently, I actually got upset at my girlfriend because

This is a question we no longer ask as it does not help to understand the disorder in the Vital Force (VF) It tends to lead away from the complaints. All that matters is the condition and its effects upon the individual on the PEM.

I wish I could give you a few "big words" but I didn't note any of them.

Structure. Here it is again... and again... and again.

she is not structured. I am tense about the future. I often ask myself what is it that I really love?"

What do you love?

"In college, I changed from architecture to art history, then I did construction and now I am an artist. I like to know what others don't know. I am an idealist. I have a genetic trait of anemia of which I am very proud. I have a history of excruciating stomach pain so sharp and sudden, I literally have to drop to the floor. I totally lose muscle control for a few seconds. I went to see the best doctors for my fingers, and the best surgeons, I have had many visits with them and all they can suggest is surgery."

He talks in very medical terms and has an "air" of superiority about himself. He appears extremely proud of the fact that he can rattle off the medical terms.

REMEDY:

Platinum metallicum

FOLLOW UP:

Pierre: How are you feeling? How are your fingers?

"I had diarrhea throughout the first night after I took the remedy. Now, the numbness and tingling in the fingers is much less and I can't believe it. I can't believe all these professors I saw could not do anything about it. Surgery was the only option and this pill you gave me totally helped. I can't get it but it is real."

REMEDY:

Continue

The remedy was repeated a few times.

SEVERAL FOLLOWUPS LATER:

"All tingling is gone; all is fine. "I was all me in the summer, I feel very healthy, I could move without thinking about my body. I feel freedom, I feel free-brained. The tinnitus in the ears is also better."

9 YEARS LATER:

Pierre: Long time no see. What brings you back?

"About 1 year ago, I woke up one morning with my right arm completely numb as well as three lateral fingers. Since then, I wake up with tingling in the fingers everyday. When I work out, I am terrified to hurt myself. There is a panic, am I going to hurt myself, or I wonder if this is permanent, or how am I going to fix this. I want everything to be aligned and balanced again."

I'll take an nine year track record any time yet there is a possibility that had I given a higher potency of the homeopathic remedy at the last follow-up eight years ago, the condition would not have returned. There isn't any way to know.

Well, we did it once why not again?

"I get worried about my arm. "Oh my god, is my arm going to work." I would give my right arm to some people because I am always looking for approbation. I am devoted to some people because I need information, but I do a good job. If I don't have this right arm I will be useless, I won't be free. I would not be good enough. This arm creates art, there is grace, and it knows how to move. It has

He has great concern...

sensitivity caring and tenderness. If I lose my arm I will not have that part of my personality. Without that arm I will be less than half of me. I promised my left arm I would take care of it. I believe in the divine spark, and I know I get pretty close to it at times. I definitely have a connection to something higher, but I never get reciprocity."

But the characteristics coming back are the same as before...

So I gave the same remedy again...

REMEDY:

Platinum metallicum

And it worked perfectly well again. This is similar to Jollie's case (see case) when she came back with itching dermatitis. I gave the same remedy to her and it was still accurate even though she had a completely different complaint.

FOLLOWUP: (Phone)

"All numbness is gone. I feel much more balanced and good with myself."

JAMES

(Late 50's)

MC: FEELINGS OF OPPRESSION

Pierre: What brings you here, please?

"I am a thinker and a head job. I think my problem has to do with emotions. I've been seeing a shrink for many years to get at my emotions through my intellect. The basic problem I have is that I feel I can't care for somebody because I feel like I am going to lose myself. I should say that that's the fairy tale I have constructed."

Please tell me about the feeling of "losing yourself."

"I have problems breathing and I am painfully worried about it at times. I have resisted medications for my problem for years. I want to fight the good fight. I do affirmations and I get through it when it happens, but it is such a burden. At night I feel so oppressed my head closes in."

Tell me more about the fighting the good fight, please.

"I want to win but I'm not beating it. I can't sit still but if I get this thing over with I will find something else to fight for. I saw my dad waste away from lung disease so it has been quite a search to find a solution to this respiratory problem. I wonder, why should I

DISCUSSION

The shortness of this case does not reflect the amount of time it took to take. Most cases take a couple of hours for the initial visit, this one took 5 hours broken up into several visits. The follow-ups generally take about 30 minutes if everything is going well.

The difficulty in this case was that he could not describe his feeling very well. Rather than spontaneously describing his feelings most of what he said was very rationalized.

I present this case because I gave the same remedy to Jollie (see case). The complaints are widely different yet the root sensation regarding their particular conditions is the same. In Jollie's case she fought everybody valiantly, in this case he "fights the good fight" for his health, for his survival. In both cases it was fighting the good fight with noble reasons but with a complete inability to come to a resolution. I mentioned in Jollie's case it was like Don Quixote idealism. Indeed, this case is the same.

outlive this wonderful guy? I fall asleep and wake up startled after a few hours. I don't have enough air, I feel closed in, I feel oppressed and I am suffocating. It is really terrible. I have to get up and I go watch TV, to distract myself for a while and then it gets better. I feel quite distraught over it all, it's been such a long time since I've felt well."

Please describe the feeling when you wake up distraught like that. Tell the experience you sense inside. (I make the same gesture he makes.)

"My wife is a cold potato. She'll let me suffer while I am having problem. Instead of taking my hand and patting my head, she turns around. I feel she is cold and cruel. When I feel like my body is in a dead trap, I try to fight the good fight. I don't like to accept a loss. I don't want to have the feeling that I'm losing ground I have to fight on."

There is so much emotional pain here. Emotional pain is often brushed over by people as I mentioned in Edith's case of post partum depression (see case). It is quite possible that his wife can't or doesn't want to do what he is asking her to do every night. It would be comforting of course to pat his back but we know that it would not help in the long run.

REMEDY:

Caesium metallicum

FOLLOW UP: (Two months later)

Pierre: How are you feeling, please.

"I was having a lot of trouble with anxiety and breathing. The remedy did not act right away, it took about one week but since then I have not been waking up with anxiety anymore. The breathing and the oppression do not plague me anymore. It is much less prominent and

He is feeling better. He should still see a therapist to help him walk through the emotional disturbances he went through for most of his life. The beauty here is that therapy will be far more effective now. He can see more clearly

frequent than before. It is a shadow of what it was a month ago. My breathing problem seems to have left. I don't feel in the battle mode anymore. I used to want to control so much. I feel like I am not in the place where I should be though where I am now is a far more comfortable place than where I used to be. I always look at the next bright spot. Even with my wife things have improved: I don't instigate as much and I am less combative. She seems more loving toward me."

SEVERAL FOLLOW-UPS LATER

"I would like to know that I could clearly isolate what it is that made me better."

and he will be able to make much greater progress in a lesser amount of time.

What James was asking from his wife was really a little idealistic and it is understandable that she couldn't comfort him every night.

I explained the remedy is a bio-dynamic substance acting in total harmony and conjunction with his Vital Force. Naturally, he was interested, yet he was rather emotional about the fact that it took such a short time to achieve what he had been working on for years. Perhaps without all these years of work he would not have been able to explain it to me, who knows? In the end, getting better without harm is really what counts.

LALI

(Early 30's)

MC: PMS

- Pain, feeling heavy and sappy before my periods
- Panic attack after the loss of my mother
  - Fatigue. Sleeping late but going to bed really late as well
  - No discipline. "I am all over the place."
- It seems like I have self-destructive habits

Pierre: Please, could you tell me what brings you here?

"I think I have a healthy outlook, as far as life is concerned but I am taking care of others too much instead of me. A friend of mine told me about you and she feels so much better, I would like to know if you can do something for me. I FEEL SICK. There is a side of me that is always meditating, being positive and taking care of things but I also have this duality of being destructive, then being positive and nurturing as well."

Please, could you tell me about the duality?

"I practice the law of attraction. I keep a vigil of my thoughts. I have my old me with all these characteristics but I have wanted to be more powerful rather than being the victim. I have had to teach myself without much support. I did a lot of soul searching to get over negative patterns but something is getting me stuck."

PMS of course is so common it is considered normal. Yet, there is nothing normal about it. How can we say it is normal? Women have needlessly and enormously suffered to this condition. It is time to turn the tide around.

I present this case because this list of symptoms looks very superfluous. Many excuses could be made for her feeling this way but the fact is that health is freedom and what she is experiencing is not. This case represents perfectly well what a lot of people are feeling. Not well but OK and not bad enough to be sick but yet feeling sick nonetheless.

The PMS symptoms are abdominal cramping three days before and pain for another two days during her periods. Mood swings about two weeks before her cycle.

Please describe a little more.

"My heart palpitates a lot, there is something strained in my chest. When I get upset I break out in a sweat. I can't believe the shape I am in. If you look at me I look fine but I really feel like I am messed up inside."

"If you look at me I look fine but I really feel like I am messed up inside". What she is expressing is that there is a sort untruth between the way she comes across and the way she feels. It is like a camera out of focus.

Tell me about the fatigue, please.

"I think it is a sign of weakness or sickness. There is a lack of vitality with a definite emotional component to it. I get tired easily. Every year after Christmas I get sick. My body can't handle the stress which is why I don't exert myself -- if I do I become a basket case. Every time I have drama in my life I call in sick at work and if I work really late I get up at 2 PM."

The feeling of being weak is rather common, what is important here is to go underneath that feeling and discover the sensation of feeling weak. In Bruce's case of IgA nephropathy (see case) the feeling of weakness is the root. In this case it is not, we need to go deeper.

Describe more about the feeling of "not able to handle it."

Here again she expresses the feeling of not being "strong."

"Physically I am not strong. I was sick a lot when I was young. I felt like a sulking child. I ate a lot of sugar, I was very hyperactive, I probably had ADD. I never did well in school at all. Maybe I am sick with a weak body because my mother was always stressed and never at peace. I just don't have the energy I should have. Perhaps that's why I come across as so laid back. I am friendly but I go into my shell as well and I have long periods of time when I don't talk to anyone."

Here is weak again. But what is the experience of it?
I think relating to her mother like this is quite insightful. This is what I call Vital Heredity (V.H.) in several children's cases. Curt's case of eczema is an example (see case).

Describe the feeling of not having energy a little more, please.

"I have a whole life to live but physically it doesn't match," reminds me of looking fine but feeling messed up. There is a duality throughout the case.

"I feel inadequate. It definitely bothers me and I feel like I am a burden. It gets in the way of what I want to do. I have a whole life to live but physically it doesn't match. I feel useless and incomplete."

Energy relates to vitality.

Tell me about feeling incomplete, please.

"I feel trapped in this body; it doesn't let me do the things I want to do. I am not strong enough. There is a whole world out there but I am sitting there just watching it go by. I want to be like Popeye. I love spinach. I always wanted to be strong like him. I have a thing about superhuman things: *Superman, Star Wars, Blade*. I am fascinated by superhuman strength. I identify with it all the time. I would watch Blade over and over again ever since I was little."

Here is not feeling strong again but I am about to get deeper.

Tell me about superhuman strength, please.

"I feel like my body is sickly. It's going to give out on me any day. I am missing something; it is part of my suffering. There is something holding my true self from coming out. It is suffocating. A part of me wants to climb out. I feel like a sad little girl, very sad, lost and bewildered. I want to escape almost like there's something better than this. Get me out, please. Something needs to be released. Something is in my way. I can't breathe, my energy is strained, there is a whole being waiting to shine. It is like there is a hand around my neck holding me back. It is like a demon. There is something about my personality that puts me down. There is a duality in me."

Here is the strained feeling again. At first we see it in the chest and now it is general.

Tell me more about duality, please.

"I am trapped, me a beautiful vibrant woman but there is a weak little child inside for some reason."

And here is weak again.

Tell me more about the feeling of being weak, please.

It is like being a little ant in a big world. I feel insignificant. People can walk all over me. I am powerless. I feel mean as if something is hunting me. I want to fight back with anger, revenge and I want to get justice. I spit some venom and I bite the person's leg. I crawl up the body with paralyzing venom. It's purple, it's Super Ant."

And now we have the sensation of being weak. This is the deepest level we can get at. I see this point as the bottom of a cone.

There is no room for error at this level, it is the absolute root that ties all the complaints together.

REMEDY:

Formica

FOLLOW UP:

Pierre: How are you?

"The fatigue is a lot better. I was really tired for the first week and then it went away. Also the headaches went away after one week. I feel more optimistic and freer. I am feeling good, different and more alive."

Please tell me about the first week.

"The first week I actually felt as if everything was worse and then I started to feel better. I felt like there was a shift, it wasn't very comfortable but I felt safe. I knew it was OK, I knew whatever what happening needed to happen."

The remedy is a dynamic substance that realigns the P.E.M. levels back into focus with each other. It is like adjusting a pair of binoculars for clarity to reappear. Sometimes, rarely, that process is a little cathartic with diarrhea as in Chris's case of sinusitis for a couple of days but nothing much beyond that (see case).

Great, tell me about the feeling of duality, please.

"The good is bigger than the bad. I felt a lot of anger towards some people in my life but I don't have that anymore. I just feel different, more alive. I still have some anxiousness but it is not so much. The heart palpitations are completely gone. The fatigue is also all gone. It is as if the depression cloud lifted."

Tell me about the feeling of being useless, please.

"I feel like a work in progress. I am feeling strong. The feeling of being lost, bewildered, the feeling of the hands around the neck and the powerlessness are all gone. It is almost like I know who I am. I don't take things to heart."

How about the physical, your period etc?

"This cycle was perfect. Urinary tract has been good too without any urgency to go pee and the Candida (discharge) has not been there."

She has improved on all three levels. It is consistent. She is the way she should be in daily life.

REMEDY:

Continue

MORE FOLLOW UPS:

Pierre: How are you feeling?

"I am feeling great. I even stopped biting my nails. Everything is falling in place. I get up at 8AM every morning. I had major problems with my brother over the years. We had a meeting and it went great. I am not annoyed with people. The itching on my head that felt like it was on fire is completely gone. The allergies are also better. My skin is not so dry."

What about the duality?

"The dual side is not so strong. I am doing everything naturally. I am smoking at most 3 cigarettes a day. When I first started with the remedy I was a mess. I remember for the first week it seemed like nothing good was going on and then it all started to change. My thoughts are a lot more positive. If I am upset it doesn't last long. My periods used to be bad, I was really moody but now I am fine. The heart palpitations are gone. One big thing I have to mention, I don't feel like people are walking all over me. That's really big."

I sincerely wish this case can provide hope for the many people who feel that health can be better than what they are experiencing now.

EDITH

(Early 30's)

MC: POSTPARTUM DEPRESSION

- Urinary track infection
- Anxieties
- Extremely tired

Pierre: Please explain to me what is happening.

"I used to be in good shape, now I am at 180 degrees from where I was. I used to eat very well now I don't eat, one meal a day at best. I also have a urinary track infection (UTI) that doesn't go away and on top of that my son has reflux. But the biggest problem I have is that I am scared of taking care of my son. If I am left alone, I get anxieties. The depression has so badly escalated in the last two weeks that I didn't get out of bed for one week. I cried all the time. I have a nanny to help so I am not alone but when she goes I get extremely nervous. I can't understand his needs. I care for my son at night, he is well trained and sleeps all night, but if I need to feed him, I end up with insomnia and by the morning I am wiped out. Because I have a nanny I try to rest during the day and get some sleep, but if they make a little noise I start thinking and I can't sleep. If I can take a long nap, then I can't sleep at night. I don't have any motivation, I haven't gone to the gym at all, I just want to crawl in bed and go to sleep. I am absolutely not able to function as I want to. I

DISCUSSION

I present this case as an eye opener for some people to understand a depressive state. Many people will wonder at first, "Why can't this woman function? She does not seem to have any material needs. What is she complaining about? Can't you get a hold of yourself?" But that's precisely the point. It is not possible. Too often the emotional level is brushed under the carpet, totally disregarded and that is very sad.

It also reminds me of Gaya's case of insomnia (see case). She was at her wits end to get some sleep but some of her friends would say, "Oh, take a warm bath, you'll see. It works for me." It seems so easy; but if only it *could be* that simple. These are very true conditions and people are suffering.

want to leave my house, go to the park and be able to take care of myself, but I can't; I don't have any motivation to take care of my son. I haven't gotten a haircut since December (7 months). I have no interest in sex; I keep asking myself, "Do I have to do this or that right now?" I just want the days to pass, I yearn for 6:30 PM for his bath time, he laughs a bit, then he takes the bottle and goes down for the night. We were always doing things and going somewhere before he was born, now I feel like I am in prison. I am too tired to do or go anywhere; we are not going to restaurants or theatre, we are not doing anything. Right now, everything is planned around naptime. I feel like I am suffocating, it's like being in a prison. I love my son, he is everything to me, but it is very difficult for me. Based on communication, I can't wait until he speaks so we can do things together. Right now I am bored. To me I wonder how can this be fun?"

Please describe the feeling of being like in prison?

"We have a small apartment; if he sees the light, he doesn't want to sleep. It's a struggle for the naps, so we keep it dark. I don't do well without light, it makes me feel very limited. It's horrible; it's like somebody taking my life away. I am confined to the couch and a book. It's depressing to watch everyone outside, especially all the mothers pushing their infants' strollers. It's a feeling of hopelessness that I have. I basically lost everything I used to love to

During these cases there is often a time when everything seems perfectly rational. Here one can say, "Well, she had a baby a couple of months ago, she feels tired that is normal and she will get used to the change of lifestyle of changing diapers instead of going to the theater." This is what I meant in my earlier comment. People can say that, of course, but that is an unaware statement. The depression is making her feel like there is nothing positive going on. She *wants* to get out of the house, she *wants* to enjoy her baby but she can't. Homeopathically, we must dig deeper to understand.

This reminds me of a story. Years ago, I was invited to a presentation by a famous alternative-practice MD at the 92nd Street YMCA. During the Q & A portion of his talk a frail lady got up to ask a question about depression, in effect, "What can one do to get rid of it?" Given that the MD was a psychiatrist, I thought we were in for good answer.

do. The bike, sporting equipment, everything is in storage. I have no reason to get up in the morning, I have no reason to look or feel good, I have nobody to show it to. I completely lost my freedom. Suddenly you know that for the next two years it's gone, there is no more of you. It's not about you anymore."

Describe the experience of having no freedom. Make it alive for me as if it were a scene in a movie ?

"It is as if I were in prison, I am confined, it drives me crazy. You can't go anywhere and you don't know *when* you can go. You are not seeing your future, there is nothing to live for but you actually do. You want to get up and run, and you never want to come back. Now I blow up at everybody, I don't want to talk to anybody, I just want to be left alone. I am in a box that I want to break out from. I tell my husband that I have to leave. These four walls will never move; that's where I will be. At the same time if there is a door, I can't go through it. Having a child does not let me walk through it. I am 100 percent trapped. It is "no" to everything I know, have and used to do. It's like someone dictating your life. My husband comes home, and he does things for me, then I feel guilty because I am there all the time. I feel totally restricted, especially when I am home."

REMEDY:

Cyclamen

His answer was "Well, you should get up early and go for a jog to kick up some endorphins in your body." As soon as he said that I could see this poor lady melt on the inside. I knew that to her just getting out of bed is an effort." He went on to explain that she also should take St John's wort. Again, one could see in her facial expression that she had been taking this herb. This mechanical approach cannot help, it is not an individualized solution especially in deeper, depression cases.

She feels "confined". Part of the feeling may be justified because of the small apartment. At the same time, of course, the door is open but she feels she can't go through it. This is the clincher. There is no doubt she has depression. And, the sensation of confinement is the meeting point of P.E.M.

I ask people to bring the disorder to motion, to life as if it were a movie scene. This is what homeopathy at its deepest level is all about.

FOLLOW UP: (One month later)

Pierre: We briefly spoke on the phone a couple of weeks ago because of the UTI (urinary tract infection). How are you now?

"I am feeling much better overall. The baby is very happy and so am I. I was three days without a babysitter or nanny and I did not have any problem. I am eating well, I have totally regained my appetite. If he fusses it's ok because I don't feel panicked. After 2 weeks the depression and the crying completely stopped. The feeling of being in prison and suffocating is completely better. I have had a lot of fun with my son. I am not bored with him anymore, I put him in the carriage and we just go to the park. I did have a UTI but it cleared up very quickly without taking any antibiotics."

REMEDY:

Continue

NEXT FOLLOW UP: (One month later)

Pierre: How are you?

"Well, I don't have much to say really, I am feel great. I am having a lot of fun with my son. I do everything and anything with him. I am totally fine. I did have a cold and I did exactly what you told me to do which was to repeat the remedy, that's what I did and it totally helped. I have not had any UTIs. It's all great."

The disorder is living as an impediment or graft onto our life.

During the first month she had a urinary tract infection (UTI). She called me about it, I recommended to go see a doctor and to wait and see for a couple of days before taking any antibiotics. I also asked her to buy some un-sweetened cranberry juice to help it along. The UTI cleared up within the allotted time frame of 2 days. There was not much to be concerned about because she already was feeling sensibly better so we knew the remedy was accurate and that the UTI was just a "clearing up" of the area.

Her central feeling of being like in a prison has been replaced with a healthy feeling of pleasure and joy with her child.

Although she is well, I recommended continuing the remedy to cement the improvements a little more and make sure there is no relapse.

Some of these cases show rather quick improvement. I do want to caution against too much optimism. Homeopathy is great but in this

REMEDY:

Repeat if needed

8 MONTHS LATER:

Pierre: What brings you back?

"I have had some allergies with swollen eyes and sneezing 24 hours after going to Florida. I've had allergies since I was 17. The eyes are really itchy. I took medication, which did not help, it seems like nothing works. My eyelids are very sensitive. The skin around the eyes is totally dry, flaky and red. It's kind of brushing my eyelids with a toothbrush."

REMEDY:

Repeat the remedy

FOLLOW UP: (quick phone call)

Pierre: How have your allergies been since you took the REMEDY:

"My allergies improved greatly after I took the remedy. Since I am in Florida I don't know if it will be better when I get back to New York but for now I am OK."

REMEDY:

Continue and take as needed

case she came after being depressed for a couple of months. The condition itself had not had a chance to go very deep into the constitution.

She has allergies and she takes medication. It never fails to amaze me that even after such wonderful results people still go to what they are used to; in this case medication, but it did not help so she came back.

There are several cases in this book where I give the same remedy for a totally different ailment. Mollie's case is one of them (see case). The best remedy, which we call the simillimum, should "work" for any ailment in one person. In this case, the alleviation of her allergies with the same remedy I used for her depression is a good example of that.

LAUNA
(Late 20's)

MC: POSTPARTUM DEPRESSION
• Genital herpes

Pierre: Please tell me what is going on.

"I gave birth at the 29th week, it was a normal birth. Now, I am starting to get pains in my stomach and I am not able to eat. I have a ball in my stomach and then I vomit. My father and my grandmother have the same thing. My father can't take extra stress, anything out of the ordinary and we have stomach pain."

Please describe to me how you are coping with this.

"I am forcing myself to go through stress and at the same time I am thinking of my father. Small things like taking the subway or driving somewhere in New York affect me terribly. For the last three years I have slowly been going downhill. I quit doing everything I do except for work. Everything has become very difficult to do and I just want to stay home."

Tell me about these difficulties, please.

"I had the same problem when I was 17. I could not go to school; I could not even get out of my home. There were political problems with the school and my friends left me alone. One day, I could not even get up from a bench. I was completely alone; I couldn't even get up. When I was in the hospital giving birth

DISCUSSION

I present this case because it is another example of what I call **Vital Genetic or Vital Heredity (VH)** as in Curt's case of food allergies (see case). The fact that a similar ailment exists through several generations of a family does not mean it is doomed to be forever. Read on…

Understanding the way people cope or how they feel about their ailments is an essential clue to a good homeopath to find the correct remedy.

At 17 she "couldn't even get up from a bench…" and in the hospital in childbirth she "couldn't even scream…" The role of the homeopath is to understand the deeper sen-

I couldn't even scream while I was in pain. In the end, I just started crying. I was trying everything I could think of to get rid of the pain but it was the strongest pain I've ever had."

Describe these feelings a little more for me, please.

"Now, when I see my daughter I just feel sad and I want to cry. The doctor is talking about postpartum depression. I feel a wave coming back and then I cry, I am very sad. I feel very fragile but I try to be tough. As a kid I used to be shy. Now this weakness that I had as a kid is coming back. It is a feeling of fragility as if I were made of glass, I could just break."

Tell me about the feeling of fragility, of just breaking please.

"Now the insurance is calling because there was no approval for something. I know we don't have to pay but still it is these ups and downs. Today, I felt some heaviness when it was raining.

Ten years ago, I was often sick with respiratory problems especially with rainy weather. I couldn't cope with work. What bothers me is that I got back to how I was feeling when I was a kid. I feel so fragile. I feel the same as when I felt with my mother except that I am the mother now.

sation that ties the herpes and the depression.

I also have herpes outbreak in the lower back, genital area and on the lips. Of course it is worse after something stressful. After my hospital stay for the delivery I had five outbreaks on the lower back."

Tell me more about being fragile, please.

"I also feel fragile when I go out of the house or if I have to deal with people. At home, I feel I am two people. I feel so separate from this kid. I feel I am weak but if I have to fight for somebody else then it is OK but fighting for me I cannot do it.

I have a memory as a kid. We went away on vacation to the beach. My mother asked me "Where is your beach ball?" I pointed to it and she said, "Go and get it." A big girl was playing with it and I couldn't ask for it. I felt the same way I felt in the hospital. I have always felt uncomfortable defending my interests. I don't want to get in a confrontation. I feel I am made of glass and just one more thing is going to break me. I also get a foggy feeling in the heat. There is something shaky inside of me and then there is this heat in my body."

Tell me more about the glass feeling, describe the experience, please.

"It's not flexible. It's not really alive. I hold things inside and I can't get things out of me so I am static. I am inside this hard cover. I am not grounded. There is this cover and I am completely empty of energy and it is as

"Tell me about being fragile." In this example, I repeat the question several times. I often repeat a question many many times until I find the question has actually been answered. This is sometimes very frustrating to people. It is at times necessary to do so to get to the level needed to accurately recommend a remedy. Asking the same question here is helping to get a clearer understanding.

Having to ask for your beach ball is a common situation for any kid but the fact that the memory stayed with her throughout her whole life means that it had resonance with her. In other words, she was aware of her "weakness" more particularly "feeling as if something hit me and I can break it. The same feeling happened in the hospital when I was tied up to the bed. I started feeling the weakness in my legs and hands and the feeling of being like glass gave me the feeling that I could not move or I would break."

if she is made of glass" already back then.

REMEDY:

Thuja occidentalis

FOLLOW UP: (One month later)

Pierre: How are you feeling, please?

"I am feeling so much better. I am feeling normal. My depression is gone and the nausea disappeared two weeks after starting the remedy. The feeling of being fragile left about one week after taking the remedy. Stressful situations still make me feel a little shaky but I don't feel weak. Actually I feel a little aggressive."

Could you tell me what is going on physically, please?

"On the physical level I have not had any outbreaks of the herpes for one month. I have some shaking in the hands, that's all. My throat became a little scratchy as I was getting a cold and I repeated envelop number one and the next day, I was OK. I also had some slight discomfort where the outbreak usually is but it never came out. I felt my body was stronger and could fight it."

Once we go deep enough, the root of the disorder in the Vital Force relates to all problems. The absolute root, the P.E.M. is the meeting point; this explains why we give only one remedy. In this case the sensation of breaking relates to many different stages of her life and situations. The sensation should not be confused with a feeling. The sensation is the inner experience that permeates through the body, emotions and mind.

That's all wonderful. What else, please?

"I had some pain in the ball of my feet. During the last month of the pregnancy my feet were swollen and a couple of weeks ago I felt a similar pain. I also had a fungal infection on the toes during the pregnancy, which was treated with medication. Last week it started bothering me again. It's itchy and it is the same pain I had during the fungal infection. The numbness and the feeling of being paralyzed in the feet are gone. I feel like I have some stuff coming out of my skin. I used to have this problem15 years ago. It is itching but it is not much of a problem."

You had to repeat the remedy, what was happening, please?

"It was a lung pain as if there were a needle in the lungs. I felt congested. When I get the flu or a cold I usually get some heaviness in the lungs and a feeling that I am retaining liquid. It is common for me. I took three pills from envelope number one and it started to improve almost right away."

I repeat a constitutional remedy for an acute condition much more often now. Most of the time it is much more effective than looking for another remedy.

REMEDY:

Continue

MORE FOLLOW UPS:

"Little by little, I have really regained a lot of energy. I have more energy than ever before. I had some skin issues when I last came to see you and now they have disappeared. The pain

She continues to be well. She repeats the remedy once every four to six months. One dose of three granules is enough. She repeats the remedy either when she has a slight sensation of weakness or when she has a nightmare.

in the feet is a lot better. I am not feeling the lung pain any more. The stabbing pain and the congestion are gone. The depression is all gone. There is no pain connected to this memory. I have had a couple of herpes outbreaks in different places. The first outbreak was after a nightmare and I had another after getting chills. Over all they were much less severe than they used to be."

BRUCE

(Early 30's)

MC: IgA NEPHROPATHY

- Sores in the mouth
- Panic attacks

Pierre: Tell me please what is happening.

"Last year I developed throat pain to the point that I could not talk. A few days later the color of my urine changed to a very dark brown almost black in color. It was diagnosed as blood in the urine. I took medication, I got diarrhea and the color of the urine did not change."

And then?

"It has been like this ever since. Seven years ago I fell on my back. I went to the hospital and they found blood in my urine back then already, but not enough to be an issue. I have had a sore feeling in my muscles in this area (pointing to his back) ever since then. There is tightness there that has not released."

Please describe the tightness.

"It needs some impulse to release the pressure. The muscles are not resting. On the other hand, I think it is connected to things I am afraid of."

Could you tell me about that, please?

"Two weeks after I had the sore throat, I woke up with my heart racing and I was sweating.

DISCUSSION

This case is interesting because IgA nephropathy can easily lead to kidney transplant or dialysis as it is a degenerative kidney disease but with the proper homeopathic remedy the disorder in this case was completely reversed. Medicine does not have any treatment for this condition and most efforts are directed to slowing the progression of the disease.

I present this case because it reveals very beautifully the different interactions that happen on different levels. Much like a weaver, with time, the disordered Vital Force encroaches further and further within, eventually encompassing the whole. When the VF (Vital Force) is free of infringement, the self remains untainted and can be used for the better purposes of life.

He thinks the nephropathy is connected to fear because he saw an acupuncturist for about a year and in Chinese medicine kidneys relate to fear. There is a multitude of fears and, in a case like this I think the sharp accuracy of homeopathy affords us the

I even started taking Paxil for panic attacks. I think these attacks came from being afraid of dying. In the E.R., I thought, "This is it." I even told my wife goodbye. I think my problem with the kidneys represents fear to me. It is the fear of the process of dying."

Describe the feeling to me, please.

"Even before the accident I had pain in the left pectoral like a needle going in under the chest. It comes and goes. When I need to take a deep breath I feel it. Fear has played a big role in the way I feel. I feel like there is a ball of air rising up to my throat, which is the same feeling as when I was a child when my father was coming home drunk. I have had shortness of breath ever since then. I need to catch a breath, take a deep breath. This has been going on for the last seven years. It happens mainly around people or when I am stuck in traffic."

Describe the feeling of having shortness of breath, please.

"Since I was a child, I have known that I have a block for not coming through the expectations of my parents. Everything happening now is the same as back then. I also have mood swings that can be aggravated in a split second."

Tell me more about "Everything now is the same as back then."

"I am afraid of hearing arguments. We moved a lot when I was a child. I remember having

precision needed to reverse the disorder.

He told his wife "goodbye" in the E.R. There is fear in this case but I think some of his thoughts about it have heavily been influenced by his acupuncturist.

He feels "a ball in my throat, the same way as when I was a child". This is common in children of alcoholics. It relates to the apprehension or uncertainty of what is going to happen. It could be fear of being beaten up or a fear of an argument. The possibilities are numerous but at a deeper level the sensation of the experience is a much more individual matter. That deep level is what matters to the homeopath. In order to remove the whole disorder, we must get to that level. This is where it all comes together.

tightness in the stomach, tightness in the throat, as if something is grabbing my throat. I was always afraid of what might happen. I was always afraid of having no control over what is happening or losing the control of whatever is around me. I used to think, "How are people going to react to me being afraid?" I was thinking it might affect my younger daughter. It makes me feel insecure to see what is happening to me. I am different from what people think I am. They think I am tough but I am not. This problem brought everything up to the surface now. I am tired of being afraid. I want to be free of that."

Tell me more about being "tough."

"It is the outside perception. You don't cry because soldiers don't cry. I never release this bad energy of not being tough. It is a basic issue for everything in my life."

Please describe the feeling, tell me about "release."

"It is not being worried about what people say and think. It means to make decisions on my own with good judgment instead of asking someone else. Instead, what happens is the pressure builds up which later on comes on as a panic attack. So when I was younger, I started to drink to release it. I want to stand up for my point of view. It feels like I am lacking emotions. Sometimes, the tightness comes in a moment of relaxation. It comes from my

He does not feel tough enough. This is a common feeling in men, especially in the United States. The important part of this though is the feeling beneath.

What is wonderful in this case is that he easily explores the connections between the different aspects of his condition. The connection between his childhood, his situation in life and the IgA nephropathy is exactly what interests me in this case.
"Soldiers don't cry" he says, is also common in men and from these masculine clichés we can uncover the individuality of the disorder and give a remedy accordingly.

stomach up to my throat and I think it has to do with not being able to express myself."

Tell me about the feeling of pressure, please.

"It must be hurting someone or being hurt. It's a physical feeling like someone hitting you. I'm talking about being mentally hurt, which leads to physical tightness in the stomach and the throat. It is the tightness that you feel when you are going to get hurt. It feels bad to not stand up for my point of view. It is ready to explode. It feels tight. I feel like a liar."

Tell me about standing up, please.

It is the feeling that you count and that your feelings are accounted for. You feel strong and solid, not empty. You stand up for something. It is solid like can take the punch. In that sense, it is a release."

REMEDY:

Senecio aureus

FOLLOW UP: (One month later)

Pierre: Are you feeling better?

"The pain on the right side is a lot better. In the first two or three days the pain actually increased a bit. The urine is also better. The needle pain in the left pectoral is still there but better. My fears are not as great. I think I can express myself a little more. I am much more open. The feeling of having a ball in my throat is gone, I can't believe it. I can breathe better. My mood swings are also better but are still there. Overall, I feel much more relaxed."

Please, tell me about the build up or pressure feeling you had when you came.

"I feel free of emotions that were building for years. This past week though has been so, so. I think progress has stopped."

REMEDY:

Repeat

FOLLOW-UP:

'I have not been as well. The pain in the right kidney and dark urine came back a little but it is not as bad as before. It varies from day to day. I am feeling nervous. I am not as good as I was two months ago."

REMEDY:

Same remedy, different potency

SEVERAL FOLLOW-UPS LATER:

Pierre: How are you, how is your back?

"I am still not well. Overall there has been a lot of improvement but I can't say it is perfect. I am more the way I should be. The pain in the chest is all gone, the heart palpitations also. The back is fine, I don't have as much kidney pain as I

This case has some similarities to Anna's case of "leaking ears" (see case). It is the sensation of being punched and, in his case, having to be strong. The family of the remedy I chose is the same.

He has clearly improved; the remedy was repeated a few times in the first six months then the remedy stopped acting so I changed the potency and he improved further.

At this point, one could stay with this remedy. Most of his complaints are largely better but what I didn't like was the anxiety. For this reason, according to Hering's Rule of Cure I mentioned in Nanette's case of arthritis (see case) I decided to change the remedy again. It is an issue having to do with hierarchy. The mental and emotional ease should increase. In this case although the mental

had. At work, everything is fine but, overall, I still feel panicked. I get irritated easily, too."

Tell me about the panic feeling, please.

"At times, I still feel like everything is trembling inside. It's shaking especially when I am relaxed. I wake up tired. It used to be all the time and now it is seldom. At times, I feel like I can't get a hold on my life. My mind is still thinking too much."

REMEDY:

Eupatorium perforatum

FOLLOW UP:

"I am so much better. My anxieties are practically gone and the intensity is very, very low. I can easily relax myself if I feel it. The weather has a lot to do with the way I feel. If I feel a little nervous it could well be that it is before a rainy day. Sometimes I tell my wife I am feeling nervous today and she'll tell me that they are predicting rain the day after. But overall, I would say there is a very big difference."

REMEDY:

Continue.

FOLLOW UP:

Pierre: How are you?

"I have to tell you that I am feeling really well, thank you".

and emotional were largely better, both levels were lagging behind the physical.

Then he came just as he was getting a cold and I grasped an aspect I had not seen before so I made a slight change in the remedy and he improved fully in all aspects.

When I say I made a slight change I mean to say that I selected a remedy within the family I had started with at the very beginning. Each remedy has its own "personality," distinct and different from others. This is why we capitalize the first letter of our remedies.

Changing the remedy really paid off with much deeper improvements than before. He does not need to see me as often.

What happened with the other remedy is that it was close but not quite as perfect as this one is for him. In Clara's case of Lupus (see case), we had a similar situation where the first remedy was close but not as perfect as another remedy that ends up far deeper effects.

The remedy is perfect. He repeats the remedy from time to time.

WILLIAM
(Mid 30's)

DISCUSSION

MC: PSORIASIS
- Facial acne
- Acid reflux

Pierre: You have psoriasis? Please tell me when and where it started.

"It started like a pimple and then it grew into a blotch. It has been going on since childhood. Most likely it started on the hands. It doesn't itch and there is not much irritation."

OK, what else can you tell me about it?

"Not much, I have acid reflux when I eat greasy food but mainly I never took the psoriasis seriously, maybe if I go to the swimming pool I don't feel too good for other people but for myself that's OK, it is not contagious anyway. At first I didn't see a doctor, it was my parents who pushed me to go see one. I always took it very casually and I ignored it but it is there. It doesn't bother me. Anyway I don't have time to be bothered with it."

Well, I wonder if it doesn't bother you why did you come to see me?

"Now it is spreading, that's why I came to you. I feel badly for the clients I see. I see them looking at me sometimes and that's not good because I have to explain. I don't feel quite at ease because of that."

I present this case because for someone with a skin disorder he does not display the common emotional aspects. People with skin disorders generally feel quite embarrassed and want to get rid of it as quickly as possible. It is a bit like Job's story in the Bible. If they can't get rid of it, people go to great length to hide it.

Bill also has some pretty severe acne on his nose, which he didn't even mention. Then he showed me his arms and his legs and there were numerous large patches of psoriasis eruption. I have seen people with far less and smaller outbreaks with much more concern than he had. That was quite interesting to me.

I asked many questions and he truly did not care about the psoriasis. He wasn't hiding any emotions at all nor was he avoiding my questions, in fact he was genuinely puzzled that everyone was making such a big deal out of it. The question for me was: Is he telling me the truth? How does one know whether the

Describe how it makes you feel, please.

"Something is not quite right. It is a disease after all. If I don't take care of it, it could cover the whole body. I don't like to take care of my body; I prefer to invest my time in something else. Having to explain it might make me miss a good relationship with someone interesting. I have to explain it to people, it is really a waste of time and I feel irritated and arrogant explaining it. Because of that turmoil inside I may lose a relationship. I'm not in peace."

REMEDY:

Sulphur

FOLLOW UP: (3 months)

Pierre: How is the psoriasis, please?

"The patches have been smoother and not as red. They are coming out but not as much. At first I noticed the psoriasis reduce on the upper part of the body, in fact it is gone as you can see. Then about two weeks after I started the remedy, all of a sudden it started to itch on the legs. Now the itching is gone and the patches look like scars. The psoriasis used to come out in bulk but now there are only one or two small spots."

Could you describe to me more about what has been going on, please?

"I feel less irritated. The acid reflux is much better. The scalp cleared up quite a bit as well. Inside the ear has completely cleared up."

person is telling the truth? First, it is in the person's interest to get better. They are not coming to waste their money. At the same time it is so unusual to not care about one's own skin that I was puzzled by it. So I asked a lot of questions and I looked for inconsistencies. I also looked at his body language. He was very relaxed, not at all on the defensive from my probing questions.

In the end, that is all there was to it. The casualness of it is the interesting part. This case actually reflects a healthy emotional level. Chapter 3 of this book shows the different levels of PEM (Physical-Emotional-Mental). This case shows a low level of disturbance on the physical and a very low level of disturbance on the emotional and a slightly higher level on the mental.

The facial acne is gone, too.

The remedy was repeated several times and the psoriasis eventually completely cleared up.

REMEDY:

Continue

TWO YEARS LATER:

He comes back with some psoriasis spots coming back

REMEDY

Repeat

FOLLOW UP: (Phone)

"The psoriasis is clearing up. I'll call you when it doesn't."

I started again with the same remedy because he expressed similar qualities as before and it proved to be as effective. The remedy should really have been taken longer than he did but seeing the psoriasis gone, he didn't feel there was any reason to go any further with it. The psoriasis cleared up quickly because the VF (Vital Force) on the emotional level is quite healthy. Most psoriasis cases are not like this and take much longer to clear.

SAMUEL
(Mid 30's)

MM: POST-TRAUMATIC STRESS
SYNDROME

Pierre: Please describe to me what is going on.

"My mind is collapsing; it's been collapsing consistently since the accident. My short-term memory is a hard thing for me; it's very difficult to hold on to a thought. I am going from one side of the thought to the other. It is hard to even understand language. I forget words. I can't speak. I have a difficult time speaking. I can hear the words but I don't understand the meaning. I feel a lot of energy in my body, I can almost see it moving or swaying like a flower. Then I have body issues, occasionally, I am catatonic. For example "Let's get up"; that thought of getting up dissolves so I end up being frozen. Most things are complex for me now. I have sensory stimulation. My whole nervous system is frayed. If I let go and relax my hands they move on their own. Sometimes I have really intense shaking. I have rushes of energy in my blood and a lot of energy in my forehead. My energy is not calm. I lie down on my back to release energy then I feel a little calmer. Just holding up a cup and putting it down is difficult for me. I know it needs to be moved but before I can move it, I need to know what needs to be done first. Sometimes I have a real urge or need to

This is the case of a person who witnessed a terrible accident in the family. It was so overwhelming were it not for the correct remedy he would have been changed permanently.

After taking the correct homeopathic remedy he has been able to go back to work and begin a productive life. Many people suffer from PTSD for years and even decades with little relief. This case is dedicated to them.

I find this case so fluid it doesn't need many comments. It just speaks for itself.

(I omitted writing some of the questions - there were few to begin with – to keep the flow of the story.)

dissolve, in a spontaneous trance-like state. It is like entering a vacuum."

"My work is very complicated by itself. I have not been able to work at all, maybe one hour a day, when things click. I can only complete a thought by writing it down. If I write something then I can say it, almost like a disconnection. It's very difficult to focus when several things are going on at once. Noise can actually hurt. It feels like my brain is getting squeezed."

"When I rest I have a lot of electrical current zipping around. If my body moves I can stop it. Sometimes it feels like a dance. There appears to be some sort of organization to this spontaneous movement, it seems as if the body is trying to realign itself. Nicotine tablets seem to make me feel better."

"When I saw the accident, I felt like I was living an impossible situation, it didn't connect. It was meshing in another way; reality was traumatized, it was too much to contain this experience. Containing it was way over my ability. It was almost as if I left. A part of me escaped and part stayed; the part of me that stayed was numb. It is like my whole being spilled or bounced out. I couldn't contain the tragedy, in a sense the vessel broke, shattered into millions of particles, not pieces. Some particles came back, like how to eat or how to talk. When something explodes, it expands, as it expands it dissolves, it was a slow motion explosion. I merged with the soundings, it was vaporization, and at the

Like a lot of drugs, nicotine has a focusing effect, which is why it makes him feel somewhat better. Keep in mind on a good day he might be able to work at most for one hour. That's a very far cry from a panacea.

same time there was a timeless quality, a hush that pervaded everything."

Describe "too much", if you can please?

"Bewildered, too much information, too many overlapping patterns, I can't choose. Each piece has a story, and it was like following the story simultaneously, like listening to many radio stations playing at once. With a lot of will and effort I can stay on for a short time, but then it becomes cacophonic."

Describe the effort please.

"It's like putting a whole river into a garden hose."

REMEDY:

Anhalinonium

FOLLOW UP: (after 1 and 2 months)

Pierre: How are you feeling?

"I have been working with my wife. At the beginning of taking the remedy I felt lighter, the energy was working through my neck whereas there was not much flow there before. Everything seems to be clicking into place. There are moments which have been about 80 percent; I am averaging 60 whereas I used to be 10, maxing out a little above that."

Tell me about your mind, please.

"My mind is no longer collapsing. Before I couldn't hold on to a thought and get to the

The analogy he takes of listening to several radio stations at once is the same as putting a whole river into a garden hose. It is a superhuman, impossible effort. This is the coping effort for him.

Before finishing the interview I asked about his dreams. They turned out to be similar to the waking state.

I believe this case alone provides enough proof for homeopathy to be known by everyone. I was extremely touched by the state he was in. His inability to deal with daily affairs was heart-wrenching to me.

Imagine the long-term consequences of this good man not being able to function in life. In this case, he is an artist. His creativity could have been wasted forever and because of his inability to function he eventually might have been institutionalized. Just imagine the costs of such a tragedy in addition to the piling on top of the human tragedy.

other side of it. Now it is much, much better. I can see the mountain I have to climb. Before I couldn't see it at all. My short-term memory is much better. I can't say that is a problem at this point. Understanding language is also much better though I have a slight problem of changing thought into language, but compared to what I had, I can live with it. The body still wants to do its thing like moving by itself, but it is no longer a problem because it is not as frequent. I have not had any catatonic episodes. My nervous system does not feel frayed. The mere fact of holding a cup and moving it was a one and now it's a seven. You remember I had a need to spontaneously dissolve? That's far better. I know my energy is calmer. I think of the human experience as a sphere and language flattens it down. Music is the best way to express human feelings. Language has its own reality, it is simply not as good."

Talk to me about the feeling of the vessel.

"I am now existing in a bigger way, it is okay to be living in a bigger field. It is still at times difficult to block stuff out but it is much better now."

SEVERAL FOLLOW UPS LATER: (up to a year)

"I am feeling pretty good. My mind is working. Some difficulties in falling asleep remain. Being in a group is still a little difficult because of the noise, but I am able to work now. At times I feel about 90 percent, so there has been a massive transformation."

He says, "There has been a massive transformation." I have many cases with severe physical conditions that are dramatically better. They are very gratifying to me and some of them are in this book, but this case really had an odd resonance with me. I felt transported through unknown dimensions. It was a dual state, a state of nothingness in the Zen meaning of the word and yet it was completely not Zen because everything was so seriously wrong. It was a state of being in limbo in between dimensions where everything seems logical but nothing makes sense. Like an astronaut outside his spaceship, I was tethered to homeopathy, my grounding and my one purpose of finding the right remedy. Thanks heaven for that.

CHRIS

(Early 30's)

DISCUSSION

MC: CHRONIC SINUSITIS

• Lack of focus

This case is presented to show how effective homeopathy can be even after 14 years of suffering.

Pierre: What brings you here?

"I have had sinus problems for many years and I am at my wit's end. There is all this pressure in my nose and I can't breathe."

How does it affect you?

"I am glad you asked. Worst of all, it is affecting my concentration at work and therefore it is beginning to affect my work because it is zapping me of energy. It gets much worse if I drink wine or beer, so I can't even unwind with that."

Tell me more, please, I find it all interesting.

"This time I got sick around Christmas. At first, the sinus on the left side was the most affected. I don't get any headaches but I do get this pressure. The thing that concerns me now is that it is affecting my work. I can't focus or concentrate. I don't have the mental energy to do even the smallest thing. When I get a cold it always starts with a lot of sinus pressure and I think I have had several colds that I would call flare-ups within the last three months. So I have been congested for a long time and within that time there have been times that were worse than others. I also had some flu-like symptoms such as bone pain, fever, etc... for several days about two months ago."

The way one is affected by the disorder is a direct result of the condition upon the person suffering. It is therefore part of the condition itself. This is the "Golden Thread" that weaves through the physical, emotional and mental levels. In this case it affects his concentration at work first and foremost. Let's go deeper...

Being affected by wine or beer is a rather common symptom of sinusitis.

Tell me more about your sinuses, please.

"I wake up in the morning feeling pressure. That's when it is at its worst. The whole thing has been pretty bad for over a year now. As a child I remember I used to get a lot of earache and sore throats. The whole sinus problem started when I was in college 18 years ago."

You are doing great, thank you. Tell me more please.

"With this thing going on, the least little thing becomes stressful. It feels like an overwhelming state and the littlest thing causes me anxiety."

Tell me about anxiety, please.

"I am feeling under pressure, I just want to run, I just want to get out of the situation. I feel totally scattered. I can't make up my mind. I question everything. It is very difficult. It feels like concentrated emotion."

Tell me about feeling scattered, please.

"I feel very disconnected from the environment. I feel withdrawn. I feel stuck inside my head and I don't have any interests. Processing several mental things at the same time is very difficult. Work sucks at the moment. I can't even do it."

Describe the experience of being scattered. Make a movie of it, please.

It is the opposite of being focused. It is like little sheets of paper being torn off into many

Notice how the physical condition smoothly connects back to childhood. Isn't it wonderful? The constitutional remedy goes way back in this case. Remember Sandra's case of tonsillitis also "started" in childhood (see case). Very often when the condition goes back to childhood it is a good thing because there is a good chance that it is superficial condition. It means that the Vital Force has not dug deeper into the more vital organs. Nonetheless, such disorder can be as disabling as any other.

"I am feeling under pressure" is the same language emotionally as it is physically in his nose. It is not a coincidence and I love it. There is pressure physically and pressure emotionally and he wants to run, an activity for which one needs to be able to breathe!

He is "feeling scattered" here is a more personalized, individualized word and therefore I have to use it in my question.

As I often do, I pressed on with the feeling of being scattered. I repeated the question multiple times.

In this case the sinusitis makes him feel like he is scat-

pieces and scattered in the wind. That's the way my brain feels with all of this: scattered like little pieces of paper."

REMEDY:

Baptisia

FOLLOW-UP: (1 month later)

Pierre: How are you?

"Overall, I am much better. The sinus pressure is almost gone. My anxieties and my concentration are much better and I don't feel overwhelmed at work. I did have diarrhea for a couple of days and some anxiety but I didn't do anything about it, I thought it would go away."

What about the feeling of being scattered?

"My feeling of being scattered is a lot better. Since I only feel scattered when my sinuses act up, now that my sinuses are better I don't have that feeling which means that I have been much better at work."

MANY FOLLOW-UPS LATER: (over two years)

"From time-to-time I need to repeat the remedy, essentially I am much better than before. If I get a cold it resolves quickly without going into all the problems I used to get into."

tered like pieces of paper in the wind. It is a beautiful description.

In Samuel's case of PTSD you see a different type of feeling scattered (see case). It is a limitless expansion of particles as if they were lights. Precision is key in homeopathy. It may seem tedious but the trained homeopath can recognize the difference in a split second. That is the art of homeopathy. To me, practicing homeopathy is like having a tasting menu every day. I get to sample all these different flavors all day long.

Many people claim to be homeopaths, but they really don't do it right. They give several remedies that don't address anything central to the case because they never dig enough for it. They do it in a mechanical way. I don't want to taste anything mechanical.

He had diarrhea for a couple of days. That is a possible reaction, which is generally very good as long as it doesn't last long. It is a cleansing of sorts.

TREVOR
(Mid 40's)

DISCUSSION

MC: FEELING STUCK IN LIFE

Pierre: Please tell me what brings you here.

"I don't fundamentally believe in homeopathy. I am here because my wife told me to come see you. I am not going through much growth, I don't like what I am doing and things are starting to weigh on me. I recognize that I need help to deal with my family and stagnating is not the way it is going to happen."

Please describe the feeling of stagnating.

"My wife has had a lot of growth. I realize I spend much of my time being fake with my boss and I am paying a price for it. I used to say I eat life instead of just living it. At this job, I actually spend a lot of time doing what I don't like to do and what's coming back is that I am a fearful person. Maybe it has to do with my father who was very domineering and mean, I don't know."

Please tell me about being fearful.

"When my wife talks to me I feel dictated to. As soon as we get into a fight, I think she is going to leave me. I was very depressed in school. I screwed things up. I was very emotional and I cried uncontrollably. I used to think I was in the middle of a shell, crushed. It was the core of who I was - totally pressured. I spend so much energy to keep this force away. It is a

This case presents a very common situation. His wife came to see me, upon seeing the results in her she asks him to make an appointment to see if I can do something for him. "I don't fundamentally believe in homeopathy. I am here because my wife told me to come see you," is not uncommon for me to hear. This brings up a very important point regarding believing in homeopathy. One does not need to believe in homeopathy for it to work. If this were the case, it would be pretty pathetic and it would certainly not work in animals but it does. As I mention in Chapter 2, I don't believe in homeopathy myself. I just know it works.

This language "growth, I am a fearful person, my father was domineering, I am fake" is another case where it appears as if he needs psychotherapy. I don't necessarily disagree but let's see how homeopathy can help in such a case.

Psychotherapy is far more effective once the state is dealt with using a homeopathic remedy. Then really

downward force without any connection to the outside. I remember many years ago, one night I took mushrooms and everything went sideways. I wanted to burst the gate open. When I came out of this trip, everything had gotten dark except for a speck of light. After that, with a conscious choice I started to rebuild the pieces in my life that were circling around me and I put them back together like a puzzle. All the pieces are making a rope back to life, reconnecting to the world and also connecting me together. Until recently, I felt the flame but now the flame needs oxygen. If I stay in this job, it's not going to be good. I promised myself I would not do that but I stay there anyway."

Describe the experience of being in this situation.

"It's like a big bottle. It all burst open, pieces of myself, and my life is totally out of control. I've been living with this ever since that night."

Talk to me about feeling crushed.

"There were thick walls. The only way to not disappear was to have faith. I never had faith. My father never had any and pride was arrogance. Faith was something you can't count on. My father is the most pessimistic guy ever. I was left without any innocence, and I had to work to come back. I always felt I was hanging outside. Nobody taught me how to dress or clean myself. One kid always made fun of me. I asked him once, "Why do

big breakthroughs can be achieved.

He took mushrooms and "everything went sideways." It would appear as if they caused a biodynamic shift that needs to be remedied. But wait! Did the mushrooms really put him in the state he talks about? Read on...

If his experience of "putting the pieces back together" is reminding you of Samuel's case of PTSD, you are right because the remedy belongs to the same family (see case). I think it is interesting to see the similarities as well as the differences between these two cases.

you do that?" He said, "Because you are easy. You are not clean and you are really badly dressed." Then I started to study kids, and I realized I was not well taken care of, not well-dressed and I started to put the pieces of me together."

Please describe the experience.

"Mostly I felt empty, I had this core, and I needed to draw these people in. I never felt much connection. I like the way I am now though. I don't necessarily want to fit in anymore."

Describe the feeling of not having much connection, please.

"You feel alone and nobody gives a shit about you. Being alone is being with people who don't like you and are withholding the connection with you. You are always going to be a misfit."

Please describe the feeling.

"You feel like dirt. I don't like large crowds. I feel very disconnected. I get irritated and I don't like humanity like this. In these situations, it feels like I go back down in the hole or shell I was talking about before. It feels like there is a glass wall I can't cross over to but people can see in. There is a fear of being disconnected, abused, as if I were spread wide open for anyone to mess with me."

This is fascinating. When he was a kid, he realized he was not well taken care of and he "started to put the pieces of him together." That is the same experience as when he took the drugs. It seems as if the mushrooms were only a trigger, the state was already there.

Here there are a lot of questions I could ask about:

No faith?
No innocence?
Not taught?
Being made fun of?
Realizing of not being well taken care?

All would have led to the same experience, so I decided to keep the question as widely open as possible to allow the most freedom and his answer.

He is feeling like he is "going back down into the hole or like dirt." This is the coping mechanism. In Launa's case of post-partum depression, I explain more about that aspect in the initial consultation (see case).

REMEDY:

Cereus serpentina

FOLLOW-UP: (one month)

Pierre: How do you feel?

"I have been feeling calm, centered and connected. I am feeling calm beyond what I would normally feel. I still feel some anxiety, but to a lesser degree. I feel connected to my life, and by virtue of being connected I feel happy."

What about the feeling of "being crushed?"

"The feeling of being crushed is gone. I feel as if there is a window of freedom, as if a weight has lifted off of me. I haven't felt that way for quite awhile. I am physically big, but I don't feel big. I am definitely feeling less nervous and fearful than before. My last job review could have been better, but it didn't destabilize me. I guess I am not feeling so trapped."

Could you please tell me about the anxieties.

"Anxieties are far better. When I got married, I was quite insecure. Now I don't pay so much attention anymore. I don't have that destabilizing feeling like I used to, I am living my life. I am pursuing things."

He continues to be well. His wife gives him a dose of the remedy once every 10 months.

REMEDY:

Continue

BIBLIOGRAPHY

- *Organon of the Medical Art* by Dr Samuel Hahnemann, edited and annotated by Wenda O'Reilly PhD

- *The chronic diseases, their specific nature and their homeopathic treatment: antipsoric remedies,* by Samuel Hahnemann ; translated and edited by Charles J. Hempel

- *Health and Healing: The Philosophy of Integrative Medicine and Optimum Health* (Paperback) by Andrew T. Weil

- *Impossible Cure: The Promise of Homeopathy* by Amy L. Lansky

- *Quantum Healing (Deepak Chopra)* by Deepak Chopra

- *Perfect Health: The Complete Mind/Body Guide,* Revised and Updated Edition (Paperback) by MD Deepak Chopra

- *Molecules Of Emotion: The Science Behind Mind-Body Medicine* by Candace B. Pert

- *The Homeopathic Revolution: Why Famous People and Cultural Heroes Choose Homeopathy* by Dana Ullman and Peter M.D. Fisher

- *The Sensation in Homeopathy* by Rajan Sankaran

- *Homeopathy and the Elements* by Jan Scholten

- *The Science of Homeopathy* by George Vithoulkas and William A.Tiller

- *Planet Medicine* by Richard Grossinger

- *The DNA mystique, the gene as a cultural icon* by Dorothy Nelkin & M. Susan Lindee

- *Physics of the Impossible: A Scientific Exploration into the World of Phasers, Force Fields, Teleportation, and Time Travel* by Michio Kaku

- *Hundreds of homeopathic Materia Medicas*

HOMEOPATHIC RESOURCES

Homeopathic Organizations in English speaking countries.

U.S.A.

North American Society of Homeopaths (NASH)
This is the professional organization representing professional homeopaths in North America. NASH publishes a yearly journal, *The American Homeopath*, and also organizes a yearly conference.

North American Society of Homeopaths
1122 East Pike Street #11222
Seattle, Washington 98122
206-720-7000
www.homeopathy.org

Council for Homeopathic Certification (CHC)
This is the certifying organization of professional homeopaths in North America. It is the watch-bearer of homeopathic standards.

Council for Homeopathic Certification
1199 Sanchez Street
San Francisco, California 94114
866-242-3399
415-826-1394
www.homeopathicdirectory.com

National Center for Homeopathy (NCH)

This is a homeopathic consumer organization in the United States. NCH also publishes a monthly magazine titled *Homeopathy Today*.

National Center for Homeopathy
801 North Fairfax Street, Suite 306
Alexandria, Virginia 22314
703-548-7790
www.nationalcenterforhomeopathy.org

England

The Society of Homeopaths
This society has been a worldwide leader in representing homeopaths. Their structure has been replicated throughout the world. Their website has wonderful information.

The Society of Homeopaths
11 Brookfield, Duncan Close
Moulton Park, Northampton NN3 6WL
www.homeopathy-soh.org

Ireland

Irish Society of Homeopaths
Modeled after the society in England it is a wonderful resource website.

Irish Society of Homeopaths
6 Suffolk St, Dublin 2.

www.irishhomeopathy.ie

Australia

Australian Homeopathic Association
Find a practitioner, resources and information.

Australian Homeopathic Association
PO Box 430,
Hastings, Vic 3915
www.homeopathyoz.org

South Africa

The homeopathic Association of South Africa
Everything homeopathic in South Africa.

The homeopathic Association of South Africa
www.hsa.org.za

Homeopathic Websites

www.homeopathicdirectory.com - This site is the best database of Certified Homeopaths. In the U.S., I recommend to only see a homeopath listed there.

www.1-800homeopathy.com - 1-800 Homeopathy is a friendly resource of homeopathic remedies.

www.homeopathicservices.com - This is the site of my private practice with much information on a while range of homeopathic matters.

www.abchomeopathy.com - This is a very large data website with all things relating to homeopathy.

www.impossiblecure.com - "Impossible cure" is a very popular book. The site gives wonderful information about autism and homeopathy.

www.minimum.com - This website specializes in homeopathic books for homeopaths.

Book Editing:

Craig Massey
MacSolved.net
craig@macsolved.net
646 265 9433

INDEX

A

E

F

G

H

I

T

U

V

W

Y

Z

UPCOMING BOOKS BY PIERRE FONTAINE

Homeopathy, Sweet Homeopathy
Autism, PDD-NOS, Asperger's, Dyspraxia, Apraxia
"The Journey Back Home Unraveled"

Homeopathy, Sweet Homeopathy
"Perfect Health, The Gift That Keeps on Giving"

ABOUT THE AUTHOR

Pierre Fontaine, RSHom (NA), CCH, has been a professional Homeopath in New York City since 1994. He is a registered member of the North American Society of Homeopaths "RSHom (NA)" and is certified by the Council on Homeopathy Certification "CCH." Before studying Homeopathy he spend five years investigating the whole range of alternative 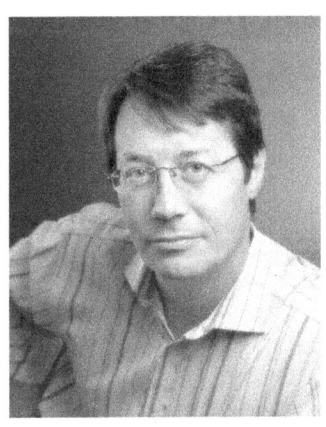 health care such as: Acupuncture, Herbal and Vitamin therapy as well as Ayurvedic medicine to mention the most popular ones. He found little satisfaction in the principles of the diverse modalities he was researching. After briefly enrolling in the Gary Null School of Nutrition and while contemplating registration at the Tristate School of Acupuncture he discovered Homeopathy. It was "love at first sight".

Pierre graduated after the four year program from the School of Homeopathy; Devon, England. Half of it was pursued in New York, the other half in England. "I wanted to have the best education I could get. This is why I did not hesitate to travel to England. It was an enormous effort but it was the right thing to do because England has a much more sophisticated educational system in the field." Consequently, his dedication to homeopathy and to people is obvious. His leadership qualities were instrumental in the birth of the New York State Homeopathic Association of which he was the Vice President. Pierre Fontaine also testified before the White House Commission on Alternative Medicine Policy on behalf of the practice of homeopathy in the United States.

www.ingramcontent.com/pod-product-compliance
Lightning Source LLC
Chambersburg PA
CBHW060614290526
45793CB00001B/30